A Practitioner's Guide to Physiologic Bioidentical Hormone Balance

A Practitioner's Guide to Physiologic Bioidentical Hormone Balance

1st Edition

Jim Paoletti
B.S. Pharmacy, FAAFM, FIACP

A Practitioner's Guide to Physiologic Bioidentical Hormone Balance

ISBN: 978-1-63337-037-1

Paoletti Publishing
2900 Columbus Street
Grove City, Ohio 43123

To obtain additional copies of this book, ask for it from your favorite book retailer.

Contents

Dedication & Acknowledgments

I would like to dedicate this book and give a very special thanks to the person who has tolerated my involvement with hormones for her entire life, and the person who means more to me than anything. Thank you so much Andrea.

I have been blessed to have had the unique opportunity to get to know and interact with many extremely knowledgeable experts in the fields of hormones, endocrinology, and functional medicine. Also, it has been my good fortune to have many great mentors, and I thank them all. Special thanks to Dr. David Zava, Dr. David Brownstein, Dr. George Gillson, Dr. Pam Smith, Dr. James Wilson, and Dr. Jack Monaco.

I would like to thank all the presenters I have heard, all the authors of the books that I've read, and all the practitioners who have shared their patients' clinical outcomes with me.

A very special thank you to Bob Marshall, RPh for help with the content review and editing. And a very special thank you to Dr. David Brownstein for all his encouragement and guidance in getting this book published.

Thank you to Janet Darnell for her very professional and thorough job in editing.

Thank you to Amy Piguet for a wonderful cover design.

Disclaimer

The information contained in this book is not intended to diagnose or treat any existing disease or ailment, or replace any treatment of such.

The nutritional supplements mentioned have not been evaluated by the FDA and are not intended to treat any disease. Comments on nutritional supplements are of a general nature and not intended as personal advice. Risks and contraindications regarding the use of nutritional supplements should be considered.

Information shared within this book is of a general nature, and practitioners should work individually with each patient to determine what information may apply to them.

About the Author
Jim Paoletti, Pharmacist, FAARFM, FIACP

Jim is an independent clinical consultant for patients and healthcare practitioners. He graduated from the Ohio State University College of Pharmacy in 1976. Jim has over 30 years of experience with bio-identical hormone therapies in clinical practice, both in retail pharmacy and as a consultant and educator. Jim served previously as Director of Provider Education for ZRT Laboratory, Beaverton, Oregon, and as consultant and Education Director for Professional Compounding Centers of America of Houston, TX. He is a graduate and former faculty member of the Fellowship of Anti-Aging and Functional Medicine. Jim has lectured extensively and internationally on all aspects of BHRT to medical practitioners and consumers, and has several articles published on BHRT and compounding pharmacy issues.

Preface

This handbook is meant to be a basic guide to the clinical use of BHRT. It was written with the intention of teaching how to administer hormones at physiologic levels and how to make those levels produce the desired physiological outcomes.

The purpose of this guide is to provide, in a concise manner, a foundation of how to properly assess the need for BHRT and how to appropriately administer it. It is not meant to compare the risks and benefits of BHRT and conventional hormone replacement therapies; that has been done in numerous resources. This handbook will not list the many physiologic actions of the various hormones as it is well established that the hormones play a crucial role in the protection of all the major organs and systems in the body.

This handbook will point out the importance of nutrition and lifestyle choices on the outcome of balancing hormones. It is not meant to be an in-depth guide on nutrition related to BHRT or an explanation of how to address lifestyle issues. Properly addressing each lifestyle factor could easily be the topic of a book itself and there are many such resources available.

This handbook does not explain the *details* of the biochemistry and physiology of the hormones and their receptors. It will attempt to explain *basics* when an understanding of such is important to clinical outcomes.

This handbook is not going to explore all the causes, signs, symptoms, and ramifications of adrenal dysfunction. The goal here is to provide concise information on how to assess and treat adrenal dysfunction.

This handbook will explore how to determine when the symptoms of hypothyroidism need to be addressed and, more importantly, how to functionally address the true causes of the symptoms. It will not debate the conventional approach to treating high TSH. It will not encompass all the intricate areas addressed by an endocrinologist such as genetic defects in the feedback system or tumors, but will provide a practical way to approach patients that have symptoms of hypothyroidism and "normal" laboratory values.

This handbook will not contain a huge bibliography of references. The information shared is based on my learning for almost 30 years from reading thousands of articles, books on hormones, medical reference books, and attending countless seminars on hormones, endocrinology, and functional medicine. The guide will provide a list of some of the more important and applicable literature references for supporting physiological hormone balance, as well as resources for obtaining more detailed information.

Simplifying balanced hormone restoration therapy into a booklet this short is not an easy task. It is a complicated topic that clinically could encompass years of learning to achieve successful outcomes. My hope is that the information contained in this handbook will aid you and that you can use my experience and knowledge to obtain great therapeutic outcomes in your patients in a much shorter period of time than it took me to do so.

Foreword
John B Monaco

The popularity of Bioidentical hormone restorative therapy has had a significant impact on patient's lives, well-being and overall health. Unfortunately, it has also been surrounded by controversy and problems related to proper dosing and lack of complete understanding about how hormones work in the body and how they affect and are affected by other hormones. Finally, we have a book that will guide the practitioner through the tangled web of hormones, hormone testing and patient evaluation written by an expert in the field with not only many years of experience but a thorough understanding of the complexity of hormones. Jim Paoletti brings a wealth of knowledge, a thorough understanding of the current scientific literature, a logical approach to hormone restoration and the ability to explain in understandable terms the hormonal symphony.

Jim Paoletti has used his years of experience as a compounding pharmacist and educator to write what is a much needed and long overdue handbook of Bio-Identical Hormone Restoration. In "A Practitioner's Guide to Physiologic Bioidentical Hormone Balance", Jim clearly and correctly describes these delicate hormonal interactions, receptor response, as well as the appropriate and physiologic dosing of hormones, proper testing and how to convert a patient from conventional hormones to BHRT.

His years of experience as a pharmacist have given Jim the insight and knowledge to clearly explain estrogens, estrogen metabolism and the assessment and functional treatment of multiple endocrine dysfunctions including adrenal, thyroid and disturbances of carbohydrate metabolism and how closely each of these can impact on the others.

One of the many bonuses included in this handbook are the protocols, dosing guidelines, charts and forms which the practitioner can use. I am personally grateful for the Thyroid Level Gradient sheet which has made my understanding of thyroid hormone levels possible. In my opinion, it is impossible to correctly and accurately understand thyroid function without it. Jim's explanation of thyroid function and the functional treatment of functional hypothyroidism is one of the many valuable bits of information in this book.

Personally, Jim has been my mentor, teacher, colleague and friend. I have been one of the many practitioners who have learned and continue to learn from him. I have been privileged to share the educational platform with him addressing both pharmacists and clinicians who are interested in BHRT as a new paradigm in medicine. I am grateful that Jim has done what was so lacking in this area.

Finally we have a book that ties together all of the loose ends of the hormonal symphony. The Practitioners Guide to Physiologic Bioidentical Hormone Balance is a must for any physician, nurse practitioner and pharmacist who use hormones in their patients.

John B Monaco, MD, FACOG, FAARFM

Chapter One
The Physiologic Balanced Approach

Bioidentical hormone restoration therapy is restoring hormone levels in a patient to balanced physiologic levels of a more youthful age. The objective of achieving balanced physiologic levels of hormones in patients is twofold. The first need is to address the patient's symptoms. Equally important is the goal of providing the protective benefits the hormones offer. Endogenous hormones play a vital role in the protection of the cardiovascular system, the brain and central nervous system, bones, muscles, skin, eyes, and most tissues in the body. Maintaining both the protective benefits and symptom management with restoration therapy occurs only if the hormone levels are balanced and maintained at physiologic levels - not deficient, but also not too excessive.

Addressing patient symptoms with physiologic dosing is not the easiest method of hormone replacement. There are so many endocrine, lifestyle, and environmental factors that affect hormone function that addressing these issues often takes time, and patients most often want immediate response to treatment. At times, it may be necessary to use slightly higher than physiologic doses to obtain symptom relief and then taper doses down over time with accompanying lifestyle changes in the patient's habits. Always keep in mind, however, that once any exogenous estrogen is given to a female, it is may be difficult to take it away. And once any testosterone is given to a male, it may be difficult to take it away. Once the hormones are supplemented, the brain makes adjustments in endogenous physiology, and removing or decreasing the exogenous hormone may cause symptoms.

Chapter Two
Assessment of Hormonal Needs

The first step in obtaining a balanced physiologic hormone level in a patient is a comprehensive patient assessment. This begins with a health evaluation that includes all pertinent background information relating to hormones and a detailed list of patient symptoms. Baseline hormone levels are obtained, and correlated to the patient's symptoms and history to determine the individual patient needs. Evaluation of the patient's symptoms is critical to successful outcomes (symptoms of hormone deficiencies and excess can be found in Appendix C). Grouping symptoms rather than addressing individual symptoms correlates better with hormone levels.

Administration of hormones based on symptoms alone can be difficult for the following reasons:

- Symptoms of different sex steroid imbalances overlap

- Symptoms often classified as sex steroid symptoms can be caused and/or aggravated by other endocrine hormone imbalances or nutritional deficiencies

- Symptoms of an excessive hormone mimic the symptoms of deficiency of that hormone

Symptoms of the different sex steroid imbalances overlap greatly with each other as well as with symptoms caused by other endocrine hormones, environmental influences, and lifestyle factors. Even practitioners experienced in the field of hormone replacement can be misled by judging needs on symptoms alone. For example, I was presented with a 47-year-old female with chief symptoms of weight gain, sleep issues, irritability, and some cycle irregularity. Assuming she was deficient, I suggested starting her on progesterone cyclically before lab values of baseline hormones had been received. The results of her saliva test indicated that her progesterone level was fine, and that her symptoms were caused entirely by her high cortisol levels. She did not need progesterone, but instead needed to address her stressors and stress responses which were the source of her symptoms.

Another example of symptomology alone not being totally reliable to predict hormone needs is the case of estrogen deficiency in females. There is no one symptom or set of symptoms that definitely indicates a female is deficient of estrogen. Even vaginal atrophy, which in most cases does indicate an estrogen deficiency, can be caused by sub-optimal levels or function of testosterone and thyroid in a female with normal estrogen levels. FSH is not a good indicator of estrogen need, as FSH level is controlled by inhibin, not estrogen. Testing should always be done to ensure estrogen deficiency is an issue before prescribing estrogen.

Symptoms of hormone imbalances in males can be confusing also. Symptoms of deficiency of testosterone overlap extensively with symptoms of high cortisol, low cortisol, low thyroid function, and poor nutrition. A prescriber once asked me for possible reasons that a 42- year-old male would have low testosterone. The patient had all the symptoms of "low T", and the prescriber and I both assumed that his level would be low for his age when the baseline testing results came in. We were both surprised to see a normal testosterone level. His issues were caused by fluctuating cortisol levels, along with low thyroid function and insulin resistance.

The symptoms of excess of a hormone closely mimic the symptoms of deficiency of that hormone. Too much estrogen in a woman mirrors the symptoms of too little estrogen. Too much testosterone in a male appears as too little testosterone. This phenomenon is based on tachyphylaxis (down-regulation) of hormone receptors in the presence of what the brain perceives as too much hormone. Any time excessive hormone is administered, the body reacts to protect from the effects of too much hormone activity. Depending on the hormone, one or all of three things will occur:

- Endogenous production of that hormone is suppressed.

- Binding globulins for that hormone may be increased so there will be less free active hormone.

- There may be down-regulation of the hormone receptor.

If the hormone receptor is down-regulated significantly due to excess hormone, then you will not obtain the desired genomic effects of the hormone, which appears clinically as a deficiency in that hormone. Excessive hormones may also interfere with other hormone interactions on their receptors, or increase binding globulins for other hormones.

When a hormone is administered, the initial response is an increase in receptor activity, and a resulting increase of genomic activity. When a woman is given estrogen, even estrogen that she does not need, or in excess of what she needs, the first reaction is an increase in the number and sensitivity of estrogen receptors, and symptom management may be achieved. After a period of time, usually one or two months with estrogen in females, the receptors are down-regulated. The same occurs with testosterone in males, but the time period varies, typically from two to six months before down-regulation of receptors.

Down-regulation of estrogen receptors also leads to symptoms of progesterone deficiency. One of the effects of estrogen is the production of progesterone receptors. Excessive estrogen may down- regulate estrogen receptors and therefore genomic actions, leading to a deficiency in progesterone receptors.

Progesterone normally down-regulates estrogen receptors, a mechanism for controlling estrogen activity. Excessive progesterone can down-regulate estrogen receptors to the degree that estrogen deficiency symptoms may occur. Excessive progesterone down- regulates receptors typically in a period of one to twelve months after initiation of therapy.

Cortisol, thyroid, insulin, and nutrition also affect sex steroid receptor function. Often, lifestyle changes have to occur to address these issues before physiologic levels of the sex steroids will produce the physiological effects to the degree necessary to manage symptoms. Other examples of how sex steroids and endocrine hormones can interact and affect symptomology include:

- Lack of physiological amounts of progesterone can appear as estrogen dominance and/or deficiency of estrogen. Progesterone at physiologic amounts is required for proper function of estrogen receptors. Progesterone stimulates production of estrogen receptors, but can also down-regulate estrogen receptor sensitivity in the presence of excessive estrogen. Low progesterone, therefore, can mimic symptoms often thought of as related to low estrogen.

- Low progesterone also increases conversion of testosterone to DHT, causing symptoms commonly referred to as excessive testosterone (acne, oily skin, hair loss).

- High cortisol can block progesterone receptors, suppress testosterone production and function of testosterone receptors, and interfere with estrogen receptor function. High cortisol can also cause hypothyroidism by suppressing TSH, blocking conversion of T4 to the active T3, and decreasing function of the thyroid receptor. High cortisol also increases insulin resistance. High cortisol, therefore, mimics symptomology of deficiency states of most other sex steroids as well as hypothyroidism and insulin resistance.

- Chronic low cortisol results in decreased production of all steroid receptors, can increase conversion of progesterone to cortisol resulting in low progesterone levels and decreased absorption of steroids into the cells. Low cortisol therefore can mimic symptomology of deficiencies in all sex steroids, hypothyroidism, and insulin resistance.

- Insulin resistance causes fluctuations in cortisol levels, leading to the problems described for high and low cortisol.

Hormones can be balanced at higher than physiologic levels and sometimes manage symptoms in patients for a significant period of time. However, hormone levels higher than physiologic will not necessarily provide the protective benefits of the hormones. Evidence shows that excessive estrogen:

- Decreases the cardiovascular protection obtained from a physiologic amount of estrogen

- Increases insulin resistance

- Increases binding globulins including SHBG, TBG and CBG

- May decrease neuroprotective benefits

Evidence shows that excessive progesterone:

- Inhibits insulin secretion

- Antagonizes insulin, causing increased insulin resistance

- Lowers thyroid hormone function

- Decreases immune function

- Decreases cardiovascular protection

- May decrease neuroprotective effect

Evidence shows that excessive testosterone:

- Does not provide cardiovascular protection, and may increase risks

- Decreases neuroprotective effect

- May become neurotoxic

- Interferes with thyroid (T3) function

- Suppresses cortisol levels

While hormones can be balanced and symptoms treated with supra- physiologic levels, long term overall effects may be harmful to most patients.

Chapter Three
Appropriate Hormone Testing

Baseline levels should be measured for any patient considering hormone restoration therapy. Follow-up testing is typically done 3-4 months after initiation of therapy, but can vary based on the individual patient's symptom response. Once symptom management and physiologic levels are established, retesting can be done at the practitioner's discretion, typically on an annual basis.

Pre-menopausal or peri-menopausal women should test on days 18-21 of cycle. All other female patients and male patients can test on any day. Endogenous hormones are usually measured early in the morning, but this can vary depending on the time(s) established for the reference ranges of the diagnostic laboratory used. If cortisol testing is included, test should be done on a day of "average stress". Once hormone supplementation is initiated, it is critical to interpretation of test results to consider the dosing regimen, dosage route, and length of time since the last dose.

- Comparison of results must be made to a reference range established to the dosage route used. For example, the pharmacokinetics of a hormone applied topically and the physiology of the saliva gland cause saliva levels with topical hormones to be much higher than endogenous levels or levels from other dosage routes. The observed or expected range of "normal" for the lab used must be established specifically for the topical route of administration.

- Timing of the sampling should avoid peaks and troughs in the hormone level based on the frequency of administration.

  o For most hormone supplementation, it is best to time the test sampling at the midpoint between doses. For example, if the hormone is supplemented once daily, test 12 hours following the dose. If the dose is given twice a day or every 12 hours, the sampling should be done approximately 6 hours after the last dose.

  o Sometimes it may be necessary to move the timing of the dose for a day or two so that morning sampling accommodates proper timing in regards to the last dose.

- The duration of the dosage form also needs to be taken into consideration:

o Slow-release compounded capsules release the contents over a time period of 10-12 hours. In this case, even if the hormone is dosed once daily, it would be best to test within 8 hours after the last dose to avoid a trough.

o With sublingual or buccal administration, hormone levels return to baseline in 6 hours, so sampling should be done 3-4 hours after the last dose.

Venous Serum Testing

Serum testing can be used for baseline testing with the following considerations kept in mind:

o Normal ranges for estrogens and progesterone are wide and many patients can begin to exhibit symptoms while still within the low normal of high normal ranges.

o Most labs still use the same androgen testing procedures that were developed for measuring in males, and are not sensitive enough for women. Most labs report one normal range for DHEA and testosterone for all adult women regardless of age. This is due to the fact that the test is not sensitive enough to give ranges per age group, so the result is not useful clinically. Testing androgens in women with most serum labs is a total waste of the patient's time and money.

o Serum testing measures total (bound and unbound) hormone in most cases and consideration for binding globulins must be taken into account. This would require measurement of the binding agent (SHBG, CBG), and factoring in the extent of binding to determine the amount of active unbound hormone in the system.

Serum testing can be used for follow-up testing after supplementing hormones with the following considerations kept in mind:

o Serum testing is *not* valid for administration of topical hormones. Although used and suggested by many, it has never been validated for such. Validation would require either direct comparison to tissue levels and/or correlation to long term overall effects, neither of which has been done. Frank Stanczyk's articles on topical progesterone prove that the tissue level in the uterus *does not* correlate with serum levels for topically applied progesterone (see Appendix K: "Selected References and Resources").

o Serum testing with oral supplementation may result in higher levels than tissue, as the test results may include some metabolites. For example, Nahoul showed that the measurement for progesterone given orally included some of the major metabolites as well as progesterone.

o Serum testing can be used for sublingual hormone administration, but levels may return to baseline with sublingual administration in approximately 6 hours, so timing of the blood draw in comparison to the last dose of hormone must be taken into consideration.

Urine Testing

Urine testing measures metabolites, not the hormones themselves, and therefore can be useful in determining how a patient is metabolizing his or her hormones, either endogenous or supplemented. Urine testing is not necessarily reflective of the amount of hormone present in the tissue. When hormones are supplemented, urine testing does not reflect tissue levels. For example, if patient #1 is taking 100mg of oral progesterone, her 24-hour urine collection will show the metabolites for 100mg of progesterone, while less than 10% is available to the tissue as progesterone. If patient #2 applies 10 mg of progesterone topically, her 24-hour urine collection will reflect the metabolites of 10mg of progesterone. Comparing the results of the two patients, patient #1 will appear to have 10 times more progesterone in her system, although the topical administration of the 10mg of progesterone in patient #2 would result in tissue levels at least as high if not higher than patient #1.

Saliva Testing

Saliva testing, if done correctly, has been shown to correlate well with tissue levels of hormones. The better saliva testing labs have used data to develop observed or expected ranges that are correlated with dosage forms and time of administration, as well as symptom management. Key points to keep in mind with saliva testing include:

- Saliva testing is the only accurate method to obtain cortisol levels at four points throughout the day, which is necessary for proper adrenal assessment.

- Saliva testing can be done on a single day to provide good representation of the hormones being produced or supplemented. In some cases, saliva testing may be used on multiple days to reflect endogenous changes in production over a period of time.

- Saliva testing should not be used if any hormone is being administered by sublingual or buccal route. These routes of administration result in accumulation of hormone in the oral mucous membranes and tissues, resulting in a high level which does not correspond to tissue levels.

- Saliva testing should not be used if there is any oral bleeding present.

- Saliva testing cannot be used to measure large proteins, such as thyroid hormones, PSA, LH, FSH, SHBG, etc.

- Caution must be taken with saliva testing not to contaminate the sample with fingers when topical hormones are used, or with any medications, lotions, or creams applied to the face.

Capillary Blood Spot Testing (dried blood spot)

Studies have demonstrated validity of testing hormones in capillary blood for endogenous levels. Data has shown that capillary blood spot testing is reliable for supplementation and correlates well with tissue levels and symptomology. If patient is using topical hormones, contact with the fingers can result in higher levels than normal in the fingertips for several days. Caution must be taken not to contaminate the sample. Hands should never be used to apply a topical hormone. Devices such as a topical syringe or topical applicator which allow application without the use of fingers should be used for topical hormone administration.

Hormones to Be Tested

For females, always test estradiol (E2), Progesterone, DHEA or DHEA Sulfate, testosterone and cortisol. Cortisol needs to be measured 4 times in one day. These are all best measured in saliva, or the sex steroids in capillary blood spot and cortisol in saliva.

Estradiol is adequate for baseline testing for estrogen status. Because estriol (E3) affects the function of E2, once estrogen supplementation is initiated, it is recommended to add estriol (E3) to the follow-up testing to make sure both E2 and E3 are at physiologic levels.

It is rare to find a peri-menopausal woman who does not have some degree of adrenal dysfunction, so cortisol testing is recommended as part of baseline testing.

Thyroid testing should be done if symptoms of hypothyroidism exist. Minimal functional testing for thyroid includes TT4, fT4, fT3, TSH, TPO, Vitamin D, and ferritin. When supplementing thyroid medication, timing of the test sampling in relationship to the last dose of medication is critical to proper interpretation of results. (See thyroid discussion for further details.)

For males, baseline testing should include estradiol, testosterone, DHEA or DHEA Sulfate, PSA, SHBG, and cortisol (4 times in one day). Thyroid testing should be done if symptoms of hypothyroidism exist. Baseline hematocrit is recommended prior to any testosterone supplementation.

- Follow-up testing should be done approximately three months following initiation of therapy.

Levels can vary among individuals but, in general, need to be monitored to make sure the patient is not at higher than physiologic levels, even if patient's symptoms have been adequately addressed.

Chapter Four
Physiologic Dosing of Hormones

Physiologic dosage guidelines for the more popular dosage forms used in BHRT are listed in Appendix D. A primary rule in hormone replacement is to "start low and go slow". As explained, excessive hormone for an individual may provide clinical relief of symptoms initially, but then symptoms can return. Once at the level of excessive hormone, it can be difficult to convince the patient you need to lower her dose of hormones to treat her symptoms. The dosage guidelines are conservative, and the ranges are based on producing physiologic levels in a majority of patients.

In a woman still cycling, even irregularly, it is best to dose the progesterone cyclically, on days 14-25 of her cycle. Once a woman is menopausal, hormones can be dosed on a daily basis. There is no scientific reason for cycling a woman's hormones once she is beyond reproductive years. Women using topical hormone administration may want to take a hormone-free break weekly or monthly to prevent accumulation (dosing schedules are discussed further in the section on dosage forms).

One of the most difficult types of patients to balance on bioidentical hormones is the patient who has been on conventional hormone replacement therapies for a number of years. Conventional oral estrogen replacement therapy provides too much estrogen. A dose of 0.625mg of Conjugated Equine Estrogen (CEE) or 0.5 mg of oral estradiol is excessive estrogen for any woman. These doses usually produce estradiol levels that correspond nicely to those of a normal premenopausal woman. However, because the majority of estradiol taken orally is converted by the first pass effect to estrone, the estrone level in these patients will be excessively higher than normal, creating an estrogen burden. The problem is worse with Conjugated Equine Estrogen, which contains 50% estrone and 15-20% equilin and very little estradiol. Even with normal estradiol levels, excess estrone will cause estrogen dominance, down-regulation of receptors, and unsafe estrogen metabolites. Manufactured patches, creams, and gels provide supraphysiologic amounts of hormones because levels are determined in venous serum, which has been shown not to reflect tissue levels with topical hormone administration.

There is an intricate balance between progesterone and estrogens and their receptors. Estrogen is responsible for the formation of progesterone receptors, while progesterone regulates the estrogen receptors. Excessive estrogen down-regulates estrogen receptors. Excessive progesterone can down-regulate estrogen receptors. Both in turn decrease the number of progesterone receptors formed through the action of estrogen. Therefore, for proper receptor function of each hormone, both hormones are needed at a physiologic level.

Chapter Five
Converting a Patient to BHRT

Converting a patient on conventional hormone replacement to bioidentical therapy too quickly can result in severe symptoms. The best approach is to taper down the estrogen dose over time before switching to a bioidentical bi-est (estradiol and estriol) preparation. Switching to bioidentical estrogens before tapering the previous dose will usually result in severe symptoms such as hot flashes.

Any synthetic progestin should be discontinued immediately and natural progesterone initiated. Synthetic progestins block the actions of natural progesterone at the receptors, but mimic progesterone only in the uterus. In all other systems, progestins produce the opposite effect of progesterone, leading to their many side effects. Progestins do not balance estrogen outside of the uterus. Progesterone plays a major role in estrogen receptor regulation. Although the normal action of progesterone is to down-regulate the number of estrogen receptors, it appears that progesterone can also increase the sensitivity of estrogen receptors and the estrogen response where estrogen activity is low. Progesterone also has effects on estrogen production and metabolism, SHBG, thyroid function, and cortisol function which affect estrogen activity. It may take several days to a few weeks for progesterone to take full effect on estrogen synthesis, metabolism, and receptor function. Adding progesterone at the onset may therefore help with the estrogen withdrawal symptoms caused by tapering off excessive estrogen.

Tapering Off High Estrogen Dosing

There are inherent physiologic problems that develop over time with high estrogen dosing:

- Increased threshold for estrogen need in the brain

- Down regulation of number of estrogen receptors

- Loss in sensitivity of estrogen receptors

Over time the threshold for estrogen need in the brain is increased. If estrogen dosage is reduced too quickly, most women will experience severe estrogen withdrawal symptoms.

Although initially any supplemented estrogen increases estrogen receptor numbers and sensitivity, after a period of usually one or two months of excessive estrogen, estrogen receptors are down-regulated.

This process of down-regulation, or tachyphylaxis of receptors, then prevents the estrogen in the system from producing its full range of desired genomic effects. Clinically, it appears that estrogen receptors are not down-regulated in all systems to the same degree. Many women can experience signs of estrogen deficiency (hot flashes, night sweats, vaginal dryness, mood swings, etc.) while at the same time suffering from symptoms of excessive estrogen (breast tenderness, bloating, fatigue, etc.). These conflicting symptoms are most likely due to excessive estrogen down-regulating estrogen receptors in different internal systems to different degrees.

In converting patients, individual response varies greatly to withdrawal of high dosing of estrogen therapy. Let the patient determine how quickly she is able to decrease the dose. Some patients may stop abruptly and manage well; others may take months to reduce to a physiologic dose. Patients that have been on excessive estrogen for many years may have permanently desensitized the receptors to some degree. Therefore when starting bioidentical bi-est, rather than start at the low end of the dosage range, start at midrange (see dosing guidelines in Appendix D). If patient does not respond adequately to bi-est 50:50, consider changing to a slightly higher percentage of estradiol (discussed in section on estrogens below). Another consideration for patients that have a difficult time withdrawing from oral estrogens is to switch to the lowest available dose of estradiol patch, which provides a more constant estradiol level. The patient can then be switched over to a bi-est cream after a period of time in which any other endocrine issues and lifestyle modifications have been addressed.

When changing a patient from convention oral estrogen therapy to a non-oral bioidentical estrogen therapy at physiologic doses, the above issues must be considered to prevent worsening of symptoms. Estrogen dosage should be tapered over time to help reduce the risk of severe estrogen withdrawal symptoms. A typical reduction protocol would be to provide half strength and full strength tablets of the oral estrogen the patient is already taking. Patient takes the half strength every third day for 9-12 days, then takes the half strength 2 out of 3 days for 9-12 days, then reduces to half strength tablet every day for 9-12 days. Then patient skips every third day for 9-12 days, and then reduces to every other day for 9-12 days.

For example, if the patient is on Conjugated Equine Estrogen/Medroxyprogesterone Acetate 0.625/2.5:

- Discontinue Conjugated Equine Estrogen/Medroxyprogesterone Acetate

  o Start on progesterone

  o Provide Conjugated Equine Estrogen 0.625 mg and Conjugated Equine Estrogen 0.3mg

    ▪ Patient takes Conjugated Equine Estrogen 0.625 mg two out of three days, taking Conjugated Equine Estrogen 0.3 mg every third day for 9-12 days, then

- Patient takes Conjugated Equine Estrogen 0.625 one out of three days, taking Conjugated Equine Estrogen 0.3mg two out of three days for 9-12 days, then

- Patient takes Conjugated Equine Estrogen 0.3 mg daily for 9-12 days, then

- Patient takes Conjugated Equine Estrogen 0.3 mg two out of three days for 9-12 days, then

- Patient takes Conjugated Equine Estrogen 0.3 mg every other day for 9-12 days, then change to topical bi-est

Some patients may not be able to reduce the estrogen dosage to this extent without suffering significant symptoms. Patients who have taken supraphysiologic doses of estrogen for a long period may have permanently desensitized their estrogen receptors to the point they will not respond optimally to estrogen. With all naïve patients, the recommendation is to always start at the low end of the normal dosage range for topical bi-est (0.05 to 0.25 mg of a 50:50 bi-est), but with these patients, start bi-est at midrange and increase to higher end of normal if necessary. Reduction in dose may be considered once symptoms are managed for a sufficient period of time.

Some practitioners will start the patient on bi-est cream while decreasing the Premarin dose. Because this technique provides supraphysiologic amounts of estradiol along with the supraphysiologic amount of estrone the patient is already taking, it will usually prolong the withdrawal time period.

Chapter Six
Consideration for Dosage Forms Used in BHRT

There are advantages and disadvantages to every type of dosage form used to administer BHRT. There is no single dosage route or dosage form that is best for all patients. Every dosage form has patients for whom it is the best choice, and each individual patient has one or more dosage forms that may work well for them. When deciding the best dosage form, the most important factors are patient compliance and appropriate monitoring for dosage adjustment for the individual patient. The compounding pharmacist can be a tremendous asset to the physician and patient, as he/she can assist with choice of route of administration and is able to make whatever strength and dosage form is needed for any individual.

Oral Dosage Forms

With the development of micronized forms of the hormones, studies showed absorption of the naturally occurring sex steroids when given by mouth. Hormones given by mouth are metabolized to a large degree by the first pass effect in the liver. Hormones are also degraded by stomach acid. Immediate release forms should be avoided as they are exposed to greater stomach acid degradation. Immediate release also causes greater fluctuation of hormone levels though a higher peak and quicker elimination as compared to a slow release preparation. The fluctuations in hormone levels can make it more difficult to achieve good symptom management. Additionally, the higher peak of the hormone usually results in greater production of metabolites which can cause side effects. Therefore, hormones administered by mouth should be given as a slow release compounded preparation.

Oil filled capsules are capsules containing hormones suspended in a fixed oil. They became popular in the mid-1980s after studies by Dr. Joel Hargrove showed good absorption of oil filled progesterone capsules compared to immediate release progesterone capsules. However, the same studies showed the duration from oil filled capsules to be approximately 6 hours, which would require dosing 3-4 times a day to maintain levels. The theory behind oil filled capsules was that they would bypass the stomach and be absorbed into the lymphatic system, thereby avoiding first pass effect and degradation to a large extent. However, results have shown the bioavailability of the commercially available oil filled progesterone (Prometrium) capsule to be only 10%. The small quantity of oil in a capsule is most likely emulsified in the large aqueous environment of the stomach, and therefore not absorbed through the lymphatic system. Oil filled capsules are not a slow release preparation. They may be somewhat delayed in their release but release most of the contents into the system fairly quickly. The disadvantages of oil filled capsules, low bioavailability and more frequent dosing, make it a less optimal choice in comparison to slow release compounded capsules.

Studies have substantiated the use of hydroxypropylmethylcellulose in a compounded capsule to slow the release of a drug over an extended period of time (10-12 hours). Most hormones that are given orally are probably best given in a slow release capsule formulation. Compounded slow release capsules can provide a steady release of the hormone, and therefore should result in a more level amount of hormone in the body throughout the day, leading to a more uniform or consistent response. This dosage form may have fewer side effects due to fluctuations in hormone levels. Also, using slow release capsules can make it much easier to adjust the patient's individualized dosage to their specific needs. Many women are able to achieve good therapeutic response with once or twice a day dosing when this dosage form is used.

The proper absorption of a slow release preparation depends in part on good gut function. If there is significant inflammation in the gut lining, as in the case of most food sensitivities and autoimmune reactions, the hydroxypropylmethylcellulose may not be sufficiently broken down and this can result in less than optimal absorption of the hormone. Therefore, gut inflammation and function should always be addressed when prescribing slow release preparations.

A factor that should be considered with oral therapy is the production of metabolites and their effects. Due to the increased metabolism by the liver as compared with other dosage routes, the oral route of administration may produce a higher level of metabolites of the original hormone. Nahoul showed in a 1993 study that the administration of progesterone orally gave a much higher amount of the metabolite 5-alpha-pregnenolone than when given vaginally, although the opposite was true of the actual progesterone levels. This metabolite may be partly responsible for some of the activity or side effects attributed to the progesterone, and could also appear as progesterone in some lab tests. The same study showed similar results towards the levels of desoxycorticosterone, an active metabolite with corticosteroid activity. Another metabolite of progesterone, which is seen in higher quantities in oral administration, 4-allo-pregnanolone, has been shown to cause drowsiness through its activity at the GABA receptor. This fact can be utilized to the patient's advantage in that progesterone given by mouth at bedtime may help produce better sleep.

Estrogens should never be given by mouth, with the possible exception of estriol (E3). Any estradiol administered orally is highly converted to estrone. If enough estradiol is given orally to obtain an adequate venous serum estradiol level, estrone levels will be too high, and increase the risk of cancer. Additionally, oral estrogens have been shown to increase the risk of cardiovascular events including stroke related to the protein synthesis of clotting factors in the liver. Oral estrogens also increase binding globulins and insulin resistance in most patients.

The oral route is usually avoided for administration of testosterone. In normal physiology only a small percentage of testosterone is converted to estrogen, but when given orally the effect on this rate of conversion is unknown. Oral testosterone may also increase SHBG. Bioavailability of orally administered testosterone is sufficient, and women only need a small amount of testosterone, so testosterone may be used in an oral slow release preparation, but careful monitoring of estrogen and SHBG globulins would be required.

DHEA *can* be given orally in an immediate release form. In women, but not in men, oral DHEA may raise testosterone levels over time.

Transdermal Application

The steroid hormones are highly lipophilic, low molecular weight substances that have been shown to have good absorption across the skin. There are many factors that affect the absorption and therapeutic responses to application of hormones to the skin, the most important being the type of base used.

As they are absorbed, some of the steroid hormones can become "trapped" or deposited in lipophilic tissue, such as the skin "cement" and the adipose tissue below the skin. Not all the hormone delivered into the body, therefore, will be available to produce the desired effects; some will remain bound in lipophilic tissue. This retention in the lipophilic cells can also provide for a natural "depot" effect. The hormone that is deposited in these tissues can be released over time, and is then available to carry out its desired action in the body. This is similar to the manner in which the body protects the hormones that it produces; some of the hormones produced are transported by carrier proteins to the adipose tissue throughout the body where they are deposited and stored for later use. Most hormones are produced in the body on a diurnal basis, with the majority produced during the night. Hormones do not last very long in the body when they are transported unbound in the bloodstream and, therefore, the body must have these mechanisms in place to protect them, providing continuous hormonal action throughout the day. In light of this mechanism of protection for the hormones, the "target" of the hormones applied to the skin should be the lipophilic tissue, not the bloodstream.

Factors that influence the absorption of a topically applied hormone include the concentration of the hormone, the area of skin used for the site of administration, the volume of product applied, accuracy in measuring the dosage applied, the body makeup of the patient, the base employed, and the hormone status of the patient. An understanding of these factors and consideration of how they may affect clinical results, allows for therapy to be individualized to a patient's needs.

Base selection:

Hormones can be effectively delivered across the skin utilizing a number of types of bases, including creams (oil-in-water emulsions), gels, drops, compounded transdermal (penetration-enhanced) creams, and patches. Special compounded cream bases specifically designed for hormone application are used most commonly.

Any base designed for enhanced penetration may significantly "overshoot" the target of the lipophilic tissues, where non-penetration enhanced emulsion bases will allow for a slower penetration and better retention of the hormone in the lipophilic skin cement and underlying adipose tissue. Enhanced penetration bases include the "transdermal" bases developed by compounding pharmacists to deliver drugs efficiently through the skin, as well as most gel bases and hormone drops. Gel bases used for hormone application contain alcohol, which is a penetration enhancer and has a drying effect on the skin. Hormone drops usually contain propylene glycol to concentrate the hormones in a small volume. Caution has to be used with drops, because most of the formulas that have been used are not true solutions, and adequate shaking of the product is required for proper dosing. Propylene glycol is a penetration enhancer and a known sensitizing agent, and, therefore, not something that should be used for a preparation that may be applied daily to the skin for a lifetime.

Any of the bases that are designed to have enhanced penetration of the skin, or contain a significant amount of a skin penetration enhancer, will drive more of the hormone through the possible depot sites and into the bloodstream. Although some people consider this advantageous because most often there will be a quicker clinical response, this advantage is offset by the fact that more total hormone will be required to maintain therapeutic effects. Penetration enhancement results in less deposit of the hormone in possible depot sites, and therefore less maintenance of hormone levels. For example, dosing progesterone 20 mg in a gel base will produce a quicker clinical response than dosing progesterone 20mg in a cream base. But the effect of the gel will also decrease much sooner, so dosing will need to be repeated, and progesterone in a gel base should be then dosed at 20mg b.i.d., or 40mg daily, to maintain effectiveness. The 20 mg cream dose will allow more deposit of the hormone, and therefore it will take time to see the effectiveness while hormone depot sites become "saturated", then allowing more of the dose to pass into the bloodstream. Once this "saturation" is accomplished however, the 20 mg dose of the cream becomes effective as a total daily dose. To overcome the problem with the time required to saturate depot sites, the dosage using the cream base can be increased initially to prime the saturation of the depot sites, as described below.

Hormone patches are commercially available that contain bioidentical estradiol or testosterone. The main consideration with hormone patches is that we really do not know how much of the hormone we are delivering into the body. Actual dosage is not provided with hormone patches; rather the amount "delivered" by the patch is stated. The amount delivered is determined by venous serum measurements, a process which has not been validated for transdermal hormone application. The amount of hormone contained in a patch is significantly greater than the amount delivered, which is by passive diffusion from the patch to the skin. For example, with the estradiol patch that delivers 150 mcg over a 3.5 day period, the amount of estradiol contained in the patch is more than 4 mg. It seems highly implausible that only 4% would be delivered by passive diffusion over 3.5 days of constant exposure to the skin. The actual amount of estradiol that goes into the body (the dose) is greater than the stated delivered amount, but it is not known by how much; and most likely is a supraphysiologic amount.

One advantage of a patch is the constant release of the hormone, eliminating peaks and troughs, and symptoms that can be caused or aggravated by such. This can be advantageous in certain circumstances, such as converting a patient who has been on high dose oral estrogen therapy. A low dose estradiol patch can be used in place of the oral estrogen to reduce estrogen withdrawal symptoms while obtaining balance with the other hormones, and then converted to anther therapy if desired after symptoms are managed fairly well. This is discussed further in the section on converting a patient to BHRT.

The volume of topical hormone applied and the site of application affect the pharmacokinetics and clinical outcome in patients.

The surface area of the skin to which the hormones is applied affects how much hormone is retained in the lipophilic skin cement, and therefore duration of activity. Studies have shown that applying to a larger surface area maintains the hormone level for a longer period of time. However, patients should be instructed to rub the hormone cream in well to increase deeper absorption into the skin and reduce the risk of transference. A smaller volume of cream is generally recommended for good patient compliance; usually 0.25 to 0.5 ml per application.

Hormone creams are typically applied to the inside of the arms and upper thighs. The abdomen can be used also as an application site, although hormones may affect GI motility. Sites with significant amounts of subcutaneous fat tissue should be avoided. Site of application can be rotated to ensure more even retention in the adipose tissue at the different sites.

Hormone creams should never be administered by uncovered fingers to decrease the risk of transference of hormones. Creams are best applied from a metered pump or topical syringe to the inside of the wrists. The inside of the wrists are then used to rub the cream into the skin along the arms and/or thighs. This technique allows for quick absorption into the bloodstream of a portion of the dose at the wrist, while maintaining a depot effect at the places the cream is rubbed into the skin.

With any topical dose, the patient should be able to precisely measure the amount of preparation and be able to consistently repeat an accurate measurement. Use of a metered pump or topical syringe can provide accurate delivery of the desired dose. Compounding pharmacists can work individually with each patient to ensure they understand correct use of the dosing apparatus and proper application technique.

Special consideration for starting dosage has to be considered with use of a topical hormone preparation. If a woman has been deficient in bio-identical hormones for a period of time, her storage sites in her adipose tissue may absorb and retain a good portion of the topical dose initially. Priming is sometimes used to obtain a more rapid clinical response. Progesterone can be dosed at twice the amount of a normal maintenance dose for 3-4 weeks, and then decreased to the maintenance dose. For example, 20mg daily is a good maintenance dose for a patient with an average build. Initially progesterone could be dosed topically at 20mg twice a day for 3-4 weeks. This allows buildup of hormone in the lipophilic tissues while providing clinical response. After 3-4 weeks, the dose is decreased to 10mg twice daily or 20mg once daily for maintenance.

If a patient has low testosterone levels and severe symptoms of deficiency, testosterone can be dosed initially at 1mg to 2mg daily for 4-6 weeks, then decreased to 0.1 mg to 0.5mg daily (women produce 0.3 to 0.5mg daily in their premenopausal years).

Topically administered estrogen does not need to be primed. Full response to supplemented estrogen does not occur until progesterone has been added to the system for several weeks, and excess estrogen can cause symptoms that mimic estrogen deficiency. Additionally, any added estrogen produces metabolites that could damage DNA.

If a woman is overweight, she may have more adipose tissue to retain the hormone. If the patient is hormone deficient and obese, application should be done in such a manner to insure significant hormone will reach the bloodstream so the patient can obtain relief. For example, the dose could be applied in a small volume entirely to the inside of the wrist or other area with less adipose tissue underneath in order to get a sufficient quantity to the blood stream. Priming doses may be extended longer in an obese patient, and may need to be given at a higher dosage.

In turn, a small-build, lean woman might not store hormones as well due to less fat tissue and faster metabolism, and may need dosing more often with a topical preparation to maintain effectiveness. Her dose should be applied in a larger volume to the thighs or another area to maximize retention in adipose tissue.

Because the storage sites in her adipose tissue may absorb and retain a good portion of the topical dose initially, not only can the initial dose not provide the full clinical effect as would be seen several weeks after initiation, topical creams can also cause accumulation of hormone over time. So a dose that provides symptom relief initially may turn out to provide excessive hormone long term. This is usually not an issue in cycling women who are administering progesterone cream just during the luteal phase, but can be an issue in menopausal women who use topical hormones on a daily basis. For this reason, in menopausal women, it is best to have them take a hormone "holiday" to allow any accumulated hormone to be eliminated. A common way to administer hormones topically in these women is to have them use the hormones six days a week, taking one day off from therapy each week.

Critical to the clinical success with use of topical preparations is an understanding of these principles and application to the individual patient. Consider that in most patients, while obtaining clinical response, we also want to build up the storage in the adipose tissue. Care must be taken that once an appropriate dose and dosing schedule has been established not to assume that it will remain the same. If a patient saturates her storage sites over a period of time, more of the applied dose will be available to the receptors, and a dosage adjustment may be necessitated. Proper monitoring of the free hormone levels and the patient's symptoms are required to assure dosage remains appropriate (monitoring levels are discussed further under "Appropriate Hormone Testing").

All of the sex steroid hormones can be administered by application to the skin. Dosages used are much less than those used for oral dosing (see "Dosing Guidelines", Appendix D).

Sublingual or Buccal Administration

When a dosage form is placed under the tongue it is referred to as sublingual administration, where buccal administration refers to placement next to the cheek, between the gum and cheek. Both routes allow absorption of the hormone across the mucous membranes in the mouth and have similar characteristics.

When a hormone is absorbed across the oral mucosa, the destruction from the stomach acid and metabolism of the first pass effect are both avoided. However advantageous this route therefore appears, it also has some limitations. True sublingual or buccal absorption involves holding the dosage form in place until the entire hormone is absorbed. If part of the hormone were unintentionally swallowed along with the salvia, it would most likely be destroyed in the stomach acid. Therefore, anything that increases the swallowing of the dose may decrease its effectiveness. The sublingual absorption could vary with the stimulation of salvia, either from the flavoring agent used, or from external sources, such as the smell of food being prepared.

Also, the taste of the steroid hormones is generally unacceptable to many patients, and even with flavors and sweeteners used in compounding pharmacy, some patients may be noncompliant at times.

Convenience may be a factor important to the patient, as some sublingual dosage forms may not be maintained as long as other dosage routes and, therefore, may require more frequent dosing in some women.

Since levels from sublingual or buccal administration return to baseline in approximately 6 hours, dose should be theoretically administered as at least as frequently as three times a day. Many patients do well on less frequent dosing, but this may require a slightly larger total daily dosing. A slightly higher dose is needed to maintain threshold levels until the next dose. For example, a patient using progesterone 25 mg sublingually b.i.d. (50 mg total daily dose) would probably do as well clinically on 12.5 mg sublingually t.i.d.(37.5mg total daily dose). With most hormones, the slightly larger daily dose required with b.i.d. dosing is usually not clinically significant. However, any increased amount of supplemented estrogen will increase the amount of potentially carcinogenic metabolites, therefore estrogen sublingual or buccal dosage forms should be administered at least as frequently as t.i.d.

Most compounding pharmacies make sublingual troches (lozenges) or tablets that dissolve in 10-20 minutes on the average. Quicker dissolution time can be obtained by dosing ¼ or ½ troche if the troche can be split accurately. Some compounding pharmacies can also make mini-troches or sublingual tablets for sublingual administration. These offer the advantage of a much faster dissolution time, generally 3-10 minutes, which decreases the risk of hormone being swallowed.

Sublingual drops can also be prepared. Most contain a high percentage of alcohol to make a solution, or may be a suspension which requires adequate shaking. If a sublingual drop is used, the hormone needs to be concentrated so the volume of the dose is small enough to hold under the tongue, no more than 0.2 to 0.25 ml. This small volume can cause problems with solubility and taste and, therefore, potential issues with accurate dosing or compliance.

Vaginal Administration

Vaginal administration for hormones has been shown to provide excellent absorption and prolonged levels in the bloodstream. It can also be used for local effects of hormones on the vaginal and urethral tissues. Dosage forms include creams or gels as well as suppositories. The main disadvantage of this dosage route is inconvenience for the patient, especially considering that, in many cases, the hormones are given daily for many years.

Natural progesterone has been administered vaginally for many years for maintaining pregnancy in luteal phase disorders. There are several commercial estrogen products available for vaginal administration. The most effective estrogen for reversing vaginal atrophy is estriol (E3). It is the only estrogen shown to reverse atrophy at small doses that do not affect systemic levels or symptoms. Estriol, alone or with testosterone if also deficient, can be administered as an adjunctive therapy to systemic hormone administration to alleviate vaginal atrophy and urogenital issues.

Injections

Injections into the muscles can provide good levels of the hormones systemically, but because of the inconvenience and risks involved in repeated injections, many of the hormones are administered as various esters, in fixed oil bases, to provide sustained levels for several weeks. The problem with this means of administering hormones is that a supra-physiological amount, or one that is higher than would normally exist in the body, is administered. Injections can initially result in high levels, along with a high number of metabolites, followed by a sub-physiologic level for several days prior to the next dose. In the case of estrogen or testosterone injections, the peak occurring following the injection will produce more estrogen metabolites, and possibly increase the risk of cancer. The only manner to imitate well the normal physiologic daily levels of hormones would be to inject hormones on a daily basis.

Implants or Pellet Therapy

Hormone implants or pellets are surgically placed under the skin, where they provide hormones for a long period of time, usually for 3 to 6 months. This requires placing a supraphysiological dose into the body, which may cause an initial surge followed by a falloff in effectiveness. If there is any problem with the dosage, or complications such as infection or irritation, the pellet must be surgically removed. Practitioners may wish to establish the dose needed for each hormone by another route of administration, and then switch to pellet therapy once a maintenance dosage regimen is established for an individual patient.

Monitoring Levels with Supplementation

The appropriate type of testing must be used based on the dosage route. Please refer to the section on "Appropriate Hormone Testing".

Chapter Seven
The Story on Estrogens

The first use of compounded natural estrogens for individualized patient treatment incorporated the use of "tri-est", which was a combination of estriol (E3), estradiol (E2) and estrone (E1). Studies by Dr. Jonathan Wright using urinary measurements indicated the normal ratio of estrogens in a premenopausal woman to be 80% E3, 10% E2 and 10% E1. The first tri-est formulas, tri-est 80:10:10 (80% E3, 10%E2, 10% E1), were made using this ratio to mimic what was thought to be the normal production in the body. When it was discovered that certain metabolites of estrone could form DNA adjuncts and possibly initiate cancer, estrone was removed from the formula and replaced by an additional 10% of estradiol. Thus the formula for the "bi-est" 80:20 (80% E3, 20% E2) was originated. Recent studies have shown that the same type of unsafe estrogen metabolites are also produced by estradiol as with estrone, so replacing estrone with more estradiol does not offer additional protection. Since estradiol is readily converted to estrone in the body, there is no reason to include estrone in an estrogen replacement formula.

More recent studies using better urinary measurement procedures have shown the ratio of estrogen production in a premenopausal woman to be 34% E3, 6% E2, and 60% E1. Many practitioners continue to use a bi-est preparation containing 80% estriol, feeling that estriol is a safe end-point estrogen and more than a physiologic ratio may provide additional protection. Most recently the trend is to use a more physiologic ratio, most commonly a 50:50 initial ratio in bi-est preparations. There is no standard ratio and, with whichever ratio is initially used, amounts of each estrogen can be adjusted based on an individual's levels.

Estriol needs to be maintained at a physiological level to get the full protective benefits of estriol and full clinical response to a physiologic level of estradiol. Estriol, a comparatively weak estrogen in itself, has been shown to have the unique ability to block the actions of the stronger estrogens at the estrogen receptor, thus it has a protective effect against excessive estrogen activity. If a patient is given only estradiol, estriol levels need to be monitored to be sure she is producing an adequate amount to offer the protective benefits of estriol.

Because estriol blocks the estradiol molecule for interacting with the estrogen receptor, an excess of estriol will block the action of estradiol, thus requiring more estradiol to see the desired clinical effects. Any additional estradiol given a patient will produce more possibly carcinogenic metabolites. By using less of a percentage of estriol in a bi-est combination there will be increased effectiveness of the estradiol, and, therefore, lower doses of estrogen can be used for symptom management. For this reason, many practitioners are using the 50:50 or even a 40:60 bi-est initially for their patients.

Chapter Eight
Safe Estrogen Metabolism

Breast cancer risk is the greatest fear for women considering hormone replacement. If done at physiologic amounts and in balance, BHRT does not increase the risk of breast cancer. Large cohort studies using physiologic estrogen with physiologic progesterone have repeatedly shown no increase in risk, and even a possible decrease in risk. Physiologic amounts of testosterone have also been shown to be protective against breast cancer. Nutritional support and lifestyle modifications can have a dramatic effect on the risk of developing breast cancer. Much of what applies to females and breast cancer most likely applies to males and prostate cancer.

Initiation of breast cancer is not caused by the estrogens themselves, but by certain metabolites of estradiol and estrone. Estrogens affect proliferation of cells and the choice of estrogen affects this aspect of cancer development. If an estrogen interacts with estrogen receptor alpha (ERα), the resulting activity promotes breast cell proliferation. If an estrogen interacts with estrogen receptor beta (ERβ), the resulting activity inhibits proliferation and also prevents breast cancer development via G2 cell cycle arrest. The estrogens activate receptors in this manner:

- Estradiol equally activates ERα and ERβ

- Estrone selectively binds to ERα at a 5:1 ratio (increased breast cell proliferation)

- Estriol selectively binds to ERβ at a 3:1 ratio (inhibits proliferation)

- Conjugated Equine Estrogens (CEE) selectively bind to ERα and cause potent down-regulation of ERβ

    o CEE also produces the potent carcinogen 4-hydroxy-equilin

Initiation of breast cancer is caused by DNA adduct formation with 4-catechol-quinone metabolites of estradiol and estrone. These adducts can cause DNA damage and mutation leading to development of cancer. Risk of breast cancer should be reduced with any process that limits or reduces the formation of 4-catecol metabolites. These include:

- Never supplement any more estrogen as estradiol and/or estrone than is necessary.

- Replace progesterone in deficient individuals.

- o Progesterone affects the enzymes which convert the more potent E2 to E1, and E1 to Estrone Sulfate (E1SO4), which is the main storage form of estrogen in the body.

- o Progesterone reduces the estrogen induced proliferation of breast tissue.

- o Progesterone down-regulates estrogen receptors.

- Never use a synthetic progestin. Any progestin at any strength for any period of time increases the risk of breast cancer.

- Correct and balance any other hormonal issues.

  - o Cortisol and thyroid affect progesterone function.

  - o DHEA is associated with the immune system, which defends against cancer development.

  - o Testosterone at physiologic levels is associated with breast cancer protection in females.

- Daily multivitamin with minerals (MVM) as many vitamins and minerals act as co-factors in enzymatic reactions involved in estrogen metabolism.

- Support formation of safe estrogen metabolites and discourage formation of 4-catechol-quinones.

  - o Encourage normal metabolism to safe estrogen metabolites.

    - Catechol estrogens are inactivated by conjugation and sulfation. Liver detoxification should be considered for all patients taking estrogen, especially those at higher risk.

    - Encourage methylation of catechol estrogens by supporting catechol-*O*-methyltransferase (COMT) activity. Nutrients that are coenzymes for COMT include B1, B6, B12, and folic acid. Nutrients that can act as methyl donors include trimethylglycine (betaine), dimethylglycine, MSM, SAMe, and methionine.

    - Avoid toxins that stress the liver, including excess hormones, alcohol, and smoking.

  - o Avoid environmental toxins and pollutants such as PCBs or dioxins that activate the CYP-1B1 enzyme which converts E1 and E2 to 4-hydroxy estrogens.

  - o Lower quinone estrogen formation.

    - Decrease lipid peroxides which increase conversion of 4-OH-estrogens to 4-quinone estrogens.

- Avoid trans-hydrogenated fats, toxins, and smoking.

- Consider antioxidant supplementation.

    o N-Acetyl-Cysteine (NAC) and/or resveratrol

- Molecular iodine (I2) supplementation inactivates oxidized peroxyl lipids.

    o Safely metabolize quinone estrogens.

- Encourage glutathione conjugation.

- Glutathione 1-2 grams QD orally, topically, or IV

- NAC

- Garlic 300-1800 mg daily or MSM 100mg daily – supplies sulfur needed to maintain high levels of glutathione

- Cysteine (especially for smokers), 1 gram t.i.d.

    o Support conversion of quinone-catechol estrogens back to 4-hydroxy estrogens by increasing quinone reductase activity.

        - Resveratrol

        - Sulforaphane (broccoli sprouts)

        - ECGC (green tea)

        - Alpha Lipoic Acid

    o Increase estrogen metabolism to eliminate estrogens from the body.

        - I3C (100mg t.i.d.) or DIM

        - Fiber (also increases SHBG and absorbs & eliminates bile toxins)

        - Decrease beta-glucuronidase in intestines, which can un-conjugate the estrogens that have been conjugated for elimination.

- Probiotic supporting Bifobacterium *bifidium*

- Calcium-D-Glucarate – inhibits beta-glucuronidase

Suggested typical protocols for various stages of estrogen dominance or supplementation include:

For females (and males) with high endogenous estrogens:

- Replace progesterone if low. If premenopausal age, determine cause of low progesterone and address (i.e., poor nutrition/diet, lack of exercise, insulin resistance, stress).

- Assess and correct other endocrine imbalances.

- Avoid exposure to xenoestrogens (plastics, bottled water).

- Avoid meat and poultry that may have added hormones.

- Check iodine level (urinary) and replenish if needed by diet or supplementation.

- Increase elimination of estrogens.

    o Lose weight

    o Avoid excessive alcohol intake, smoking, and trans-hydrogenated fats

    o Probiotic

        ▪ May take Calcium-D-Glucarate for 1-2 months

    o I3C and/or DIM

    o Liver Detox program (one week up to one month)

    o Daily MVM

    o Increase fiber intake

    o Antioxidant supplementation

        ▪ Combination of at least two antioxidants, one of which should be NAC or resveratrol

For all women who want to supplement estrogen:

- Progesterone restored to physiologic levels

- Assess and treat other sex and endocrine hormone imbalances

- Liver detox program—at least 7-day program

- Daily MVM

- Probiotic daily for at least two months

- I would also encourage:

  o Methylation support (B1, B6, B12, folate, and methyl donor)

  o Antioxidant supplementation

    ▪ Combination of at least two antioxidants, one of which should be NAC or resveratrol

For women at high risk (family history, overweight, no children, smokers, etc):

- Progesterone restored to physiologic levels

- Assess and treat other sex and endocrine hormone imbalances

- Check iodine level (urinary) and replenish if needed by diet or supplementation

- Liver detox program - 28 day

- Avoid excessive alcohol intake and smoking

- Avoid trans-hydrogenated fats, pollutants, toxins, xenoestrogens

- Daily MVM

- Probiotic daily

- Methylation support (B1, B6, B12, folate, and methyl donor)

- Antioxidant supplementation

  o Combination of at least three antioxidants

  ▪ NAC, resveratrol and either Vitamin C, Vitamin E, or Alpha Lipoic Acid

- Moderate exercise at least 4 times a week

- Encourage consumption of green tea or supplement ECGC

- Glutathione 1-2 grams daily

The 2OH:16OH Ratio Theory:

For years, most practitioners that practiced natural or bioidentical hormone replacement were taught that the ratio of 2-hydroxyestrone to 16-hydroxyestrone was correlated to breast cancer risk. *In vitro* studies showed a lower 2:16 ratio linked to increased risk. However, no *in vivo* study has actually demonstrated there was an increased risk. The studies that claimed there was a correlation failed to look at the possible involvement of 4-hydroxy estrogens and their influence on the risk. We now know that the 4-OH estrogens are the metabolites that form quinone metabolites that can damage DNA, and perhaps breast cancer risk is correlated to a 2:4 OH ratio. Additionally, there are more numerous studies that fail to demonstrate any correlation, so at best the theory that raising the 2:1 ratio decreased breast cancer risk is controversial. The 2-OH and 16-OH estrone metabolites were determined by 24 urine measurements, and much of the education on the subject was taught by persons with financial interest in urine testing labs or nutritional products that increased the ratio. Cavalieri, Rogan, and others have done work showing (1) the estrogen metabolites are produced from estradiol as well as estrone and (2) 16-OH estrogens are protein bound and have no further effect. 16-OH-estrone is a potent estrogen and can cause proliferation of breast cells, but does not form DNA adducts that initiate cancer. Administration of I3C or DIM will raise the ratio of 2:16-OH estrogens as well as increase overall elimination of estrogens. Although this is beneficial, it does not necessarily decrease breast cancer risk by changing the 2:16-OH estrogen ratio. The above suggestions can modify risk, and without the added expense of measuring the four metabolites of estrogen.

Breast cancer risk should always be thoroughly discussed with the patient, and some outline for preventative strategies provided. Differences in risk associated with conventional hormone therapies vs. physiological use of bioidentical hormones should be shared.

Chapter Nine
Assessment and Treatment
of Adrenal Dysfunction

The causes of stress are abundant, and the long term consequences on patient health of untreated adrenal dysfunction are extensive. Effects of stress are cumulative and additive over time. Therefore, numerous patients experience some degree of adrenal dysfunction to the point where symptoms are present, and symptoms of other hormonal imbalances are worsened.

Assessment of adrenal function starts with the patient's symptoms (see "Cortisol Symptoms in Appendix C). Patients that exhibit a significant number of symptoms listed under excess and deficient cortisol are almost always are suffering from some degree of adrenal dysfunction. Many patients seeking hormonal replacement exhibit common adrenal dysfunction symptoms of fatigue, weight gain, sleep disturbances, memory issues, stress sensitivity, depression, food cravings, etc. Management of these symptoms requires adequate assessment of cortisol levels as well as the sex steroids to determine the causes.

Proper assessment and individualized treatment of adrenal dysfunction requires cortisol measurement in saliva at least four times in a day. Since symptoms of adrenal dysfunction overlap extensively with symptoms of other hormone imbalances, a basic baseline assessment of adrenal status can be qualitatively judged by questionnaire or lifestyle diary to establish a need to test. In Dr. James Wilson's book, Adrenal Fatigue: The 21st Century Stress Syndrome, there is an 11-page questionnaire that can used to evaluate overall adrenal status. A questionnaire may help convince a patient there is an issue with their adrenal glands, but it does not take into account an individual's daily response. Patients may be stressed and have fluctuations in their cortisol levels at different times of the day based on their individual life situations.

Fluctuations in cortisol will cause energy, sleep, and dietary patterns that can be used to recognize adrenal dysfunction. High cortisol levels will result in energy but less appetite and interference with sleep. Low cortisol results in low energy, difficulty awakening and being alert, and mid-day crashes in energy. Low cortisol creates cravings for salt and for stimulating substances including caffeine, nicotine, sugar, and carbohydrates. A manner that can aid in evaluating adrenal status is to have the patient keep a dairy for three days in which they:

- Record their energy level on a basis of 1 to 10 at least every two hours

  o Record any time they notice highs and lows of energy

- Record time and intake of food and beverages, nicotine, caffeine, and drugs

- Record any times they feel they should be sleeping and are not

    o Indicate whether their mind is stimulated and active or sluggish

- Record any naps and hours slept at night

A pattern of low energy followed by consuming stimulation substances (caffeine, nicotine, sugar, carbohydrates) which replenish energy indicates low adrenal cortisol in most cases. Poor sleep can indicate high cortisol, but may also be caused by chronic hypocortisolism.

Cortisol can be considered the regulator or the ruler of the hormones. High cortisol levels interfere with the actions of the sex steroids, so symptoms include those for deficiency in estrogen, progesterone, and testosterone. High cortisol also suppresses TSH, inhibits conversion of T4 to the active T3, and lowers thyroid receptor response. High cortisol inhibits growth hormone and stimulates visceral fat deposition and high insulin, leading to metabolic syndrome. Cortisol stimulates aromatase which converts testosterone to estrogen. Prolonged hypercortisolism leads to degeneration of the hippocampus, hypothalamus, pre-frontal cortex, and amygdala, causing symptoms from memory issues to depression to emotional instability.

Low cortisol can result in reduced cellular absorption of hormones, reduced density of hormone receptors, reduced thyroid receptor response, and low pregnenolone, progesterone, and aldosterone due to alterations in the steroidogenic pathways.

Unless cortisol is adequately assessed and adrenal dysfunction properly treated, many of the symptoms patients are wishing to manage with hormone replacement will never be adequately addressed with sex steroid restoration alone. Since stress and adrenal dysfunction are so common, testing cortisol as well as the sex steroids should be included on baseline testing for most if not all patients of both sexes.

Cortisol should be measured in saliva. Patients should be asked to test their cortisol on an "average" day of stress.

Urine testing (24-hour collection) is helpful in indicating cortisol reserve, but does not allow evaluation of individual cortisol fluctuations throughout the day, and may underestimate cortisol levels in up to 30% of patients. A patient with high morning and high night cortisol but low cortisol throughout the day could have the same total daily cortisol output as a person that had normal levels all day. Serum cortisol assays are limited as to the times and number of measurements in a day, can be highly variable due to cortisol binding globulin, and suffer from considerable inaccuracies which lead to overestimated levels by an average of 70% in 44-56% of patients.

Treatment of adrenal dysfunction is based on the patient's cortisol production throughout the day, so testing in salvia at least four times throughout the day provides the best information for individualizing treatment. A morning cortisol level alone is not very helpful, as treatment is based on how the level varies the rest of the day. Even a two point cortisol (a.m. and p.m.) lacks information and can be misleading in that a patient could be high or normal for both tests, but below normal during the day.

Testosterone and DHEA

When the adrenal glands are chronically stressed and cortisol levels are elevated, testosterone and DHEA levels rise along with them. This increase in androgens may be the result of increased production due to stimulation, and/or the brain attempting to offset the genomic actions of high cortisol with opposite genomic actions of the androgens. With continued stress, adrenal cortisol reserves and output cannot keep up with demand, and cortisol levels begin to fall. Testosterone and DHEA levels fall along with the declining cortisol levels. *Which levels decline first and in what order is highly individual.*

A common pattern of progression in adrenal dysfunction is one in which cortisol levels remain high in the morning and at night, with low or low normal levels during the day. Often the night cortisol level then drops, with only the morning cortisol remaining elevated. Eventually the morning cortisol drops to a normal level, then to low. The levels of androgens usually begin to decline when cortisol levels first begin to fall. Low cortisol at one or more points in a day, along with low androgens, especially DHEA, indicates adrenal insufficiency.

Some patients may exhibit signs and symptoms of both high and low cortisol but their 4-point saliva cortisol test results in a fairly normal pattern. The previous high cortisol levels have fallen evenly throughout the entire day and create a fairly normal pattern. In these patients, assessment of the cortisol pattern alone would not provide a reflection of the clinical symptoms, but evaluation of the androgen levels will almost always reflect a deficient status, indicating adrenal dysfunction.

Chronic low cortisol may also lower pregnenolone and progesterone levels. Prolonged elevations in ACTH and cortisol cause circulatory changes in the adrenal glands which result in an increased production of cortisol and reduction in the amounts of aldosterone and progesterone normally produced. Clinical manifestations include estrogen dominance symptoms and blood volume/pressure issues.

Always attempt to identify and treat the *underlying cause* of abnormal cortisol patterns. Treatment modalities for adrenal function include:

- Vitamin and Mineral Support

- Methyl Donors

- Adaptogens

- Theanine

- Phosphatidylserine

- 5-Hydroxytryptophan (5HTP)

- Glandular Extracts

- Hydrocortisone

- Endocrine Hormones

- Sleep Enhancement

- Lifestyle Modifications

- Dietary Adjustments

Vitamin and Mineral Support

The adrenal glands use and demand more nutritional support than most if not all other glands in the body. Continual and repeated stress increases the nutritional support needed for the adrenal glands. Patients that have been or presently are significantly stressed should consider taking a vitamin/mineral combination made specifically for adrenal health. This would be in addition to a daily MVM for general health purposes. Even after adrenal health is re-established, taking a vitamin/mineral to support the adrenals would be appropriate in times of stress.

Vitamins and minerals for adrenal support include:

- Vitamin C   2-5 grams daily

- Magnesium Glycinate   300-600mg daily in divided doses for relaxation and 400-800 mg before bedtime to help with sleep

- B Vitamins   Super B complex daily and additional Pantothenic Acid (B5) up to 1.5 grams daily total

- Selenium   200mcg daily

- Zinc   25-50 mg daily

- Calcium   400-800 mg daily

- Vitamin E with mixed tocopherols   800 IU daily

- Copper, Sodium, Manganese

Methyl Donors

If there is a scarcity of methyl donors, epinephrine synthesis from norepinephrine will be deficient. Cortisol will rise in an attempt to increase epinephrine receptor synthesis. Methyl donors include:

- MSM   500-1000 mg daily
- Trimethylglycine   500-1000 mg daily
- Dimethylglycine.   250-500 mg daily
- Methionine   500-1000 mg daily
- SAMe   200-400 mg b.i.d.

Adaptogens

Adaptogens are plant-based compounds that increase the ability of an organism to adapt to environmental factors and to avoid damage from such factors. They promote cellular resistance to stress and help maintain an adaptive state of homeostasis. They act by agonistic action on HPA axis regulation, stimulate the nervous system by regulating elements of the stress response and modulating stimulus-response coupling, and control key mediators of stress including cortisol and nitric oxide. Examples of adaptogens include ashwagandha, rhodiola, Siberian ginseng, maca, relora, schisandra, licorice, holy basil, cordyceps, astragalus, bacopa, and several others.

Ashwagandha (*Withania somnifera*): Helps control cortisol levels, reduce fatigue, produce better sleep, create a sense of wellbeing, and provides anti-anxiety and neuroprotective effects. Also helps stimulate thyroid function and has cardioprotective and immunnomodulatory benefits. Typical dose is 3 to 6 grams daily, with up to 10 grams for occasional acute stress. Caution: large amounts are contraindicated in pregnancy, so not more than 1/2 to 1 tsp. of the powder should be taken daily if possibly pregnant.

Rhodiola (*Rhodiola rosea*): Prevents stress induced adrenal catecholamine depletion and improves physical endurance. Dosed at 250 mg (3-5% rosavin & 1-3% salidroside) 1-3 times daily.

Siberian Ginseng (*Eleutherococcus senticosus*): Delays the exhaustive phase of the stress reaction and prevents depletion of corticosteroids and epinephrine. Boosts energy, increases physical and mental performance, extends endurance, and improves tolerance of environmental stimuli. Typical dose of dried root is 2-8 grams daily; fluid extract is 2-6 ml 1-3 times daily.

Maca (*Lepidium meyenii*): Eliminates variations in homeostasis induced by stress, reduces stress induced adrenal hyperplasia and reduces corticosterone levels. Dosed 5-10 grams b.i.d. dried powder.

Relora®: Proprietary blend of *Magnolia officinalis* and *Phellodendron amurense* (bark). Marketed for stress-related appetite control and reduction of stress-related fat deposition. Claimed to have anti-anxiety and anti-depressant properties. Lack of studies to support claims, but reports of good clinical outcomes. Dose is 250mg t.i.d. May cause headaches, drowsiness, and foggy feeling.

Schisandra (*Schisandra chinensis*): Helps regulate levels of cortisol and nitric oxide. Increases physical work capacity and endurance. Improves mental function and reduces fatigue after physical exercise. Recommended doses of schisandra are 1.5–15 g of dried fruit daily, 2–4 ml of tincture three times daily, 1.5–6 g of powder daily, one to three cups of tea once daily, or 1.5 g in capsule form daily.

Licorice (*Glycyrrhiza glabra*): blocks conversion of cortisol into cortisone and has mineralocorticoid and glucocorticoid activity. Dose at 200-300 mg of licorice glycyrrhiza daily. Caution: do not use in patients with high blood pressure.

Holy Basil (*Ocimum sanctum*): modulates adrenal corticosterone levels, decreases recovery time from stress and may protect against stress-induced immune alterations. Dose is 400-800 mg b.i.d standardized to 1% ursolic acid.

Cordyceps (*Cordyceps sinensis*): Properties similar to ginseng. Decreases fatigue, enhances stamina, increases energy, and stimulates the immune system. Typical dose is 3 grams daily.

Astragalus (*Astragalus membranaceus*): stimulates immune system.

Used to facilitate the body's normal response to occasional stress and promote a healthy response to environmental stress. Stimulates immune system, has anti-oxidant and anti-viral properties, and may boost production of telomerase.

Standardized extract: 250-500 mg, three to four times a day, standardized to 0.4% 4-hydroxy-3-methoxy isoflavone 7-sug. Powdered root: 500 - 1,000 mg, three or four times per day

Bacopa (*Bacopa monnieri*): Beneficial effects on anxiety as well as mental fatigue. CNS effects believed to be GABAergic system mediated. May affect serotonin and norepinephrine levels. Typical dose is 300mg daily.

No one can predict which adaptogens(s) will work best for any individual. As a single use agent, ashwagandha is among the best choices, but in most all cases it might be best to use a combination adaptogen product that contains 3 or more agents, including ashwagandha. If patient needs to take for longer than 3-4 months, consider switching to a different adaptogen or combination.

Caution: although adaptogens are generally safe and very well tolerated, always check for medication interactions and contraindications before using.

Theanine

Amino acid extracted from green tea. Exerts anti-stress effects during acute stress. Enhances brain alpha wave activity for relaxation. Influences the secretion and function of serotonin and dopamine. May use 100-200mg 2-3 times a day for relaxation and 100-300 mg 30 to 60 minutes before bedtime to aid getting to sleep.

Phosphatidylserine (PS)

Dampens stress induced ACTH and cortisol release. Induces release of acetylcholine, dopamine, and norepinephrine. Improves stress resistance to acute stressor. Improves mood, helps prevent chronic stress-induced memory loss.

100-800 mg daily in divided doses. 300 mg in the evening to suppress nighttime cortisol and help induce sleep.

Note: Effects of PS wear off with time in some patients. Patients should be cautioned that PS is a temporary crutch to help while they make the necessary lifestyle modifications, and if the effects wear off, there may not be another agent to substitute.

Caution: If a patient has high nighttime and/or morning cortisol levels, but has low to low normal daytime levels, PS may suppress cortisol to the point that the daytime levels are also lowered, causing extreme fatigue.

5-Hydroxytryptophan (5HTP)

Precursor to serotonin and melatonin. May help with carbohydrate cravings and sleep. 50-150 mg before meals and 150-300mg before bedtime.

Glandular Extracts

Glandular extracts come from the hormone-producing glands of animals, usually cows, but sometimes sheep and pigs. They contain dried and ground-up raw animal glandular tissues or extracts of those tissues - from the thyroid, thymus, adrenals, pituitary, ovaries, testis, and pancreas. Glandulars are used to rebuild the strength of the gland. Although not a requirement for recovery from adrenal dysfunction, glandulars speed of the process of recovery significantly. A raw adrenal extract can be used, or a multi-glandular extract containing extracts from adrenal, hypothalamus, pituitary, and thyroid glands, may be preferred to support the entire HPA axis. Adrenal glandular extracts do contain small amounts of cortisone and other adrenal hormones. They may also contain peptides which promote endogenous adrenal hormone production. Dosage is usually 1-6 capsules daily in divided doses, and varies with product, severity of symptoms, and degree of hypocortisolism. Recommendation is to use glandulars for any patient who has two or more cortisol levels below normal, and/or is too fatigued to function adequately during the day.

Hydrocortisone

Hydrocortisone can be supplemented when cortisol levels are low and patient is fatigued to the point they cannot function adequately to make recommended lifestyle changes. Caution should be taken in considering supplementing hydrocortisone. The patient became adrenally insufficient after years of sustaining a high cortisol level, during which energy levels were good, and general complaints usually less. Some patients will feel better on hydrocortisone and might not be encouraged to make necessary lifestyle changes. Hydrocortisone supplementation should be considered a crutch, to help the patient until they can obtain normal adrenal strength. Doses used are commonly 5-30 mg daily, in immediate release or slow released preparations. Immediate release preparations may present problems in some patients. As the level of cortisol drops 4-6 hours after the dose, the patient may experience severe food cravings and/or low energy, and may be tempted to dose the hydrocortisone more often than prescribed. Dosage should be based on the individual's cortisol levels and energy ratings. Some patients may do well on a morning dose alone, others may have to add a dose at noon, and some may even require a late afternoon dose. Dose should be reduced later in the day.

Typical dosing schedules:

- 5 to 15 mg in a.m. (IR)   OR • 10-30 mg (SR) in a.m.   OR • 5-10 mg (SR) in the a.m.

- 5 to 10 mg at noon   • 2.5 -5 mg (SR) at noon

- 2.5 to 5 mg late afternoon

If a patient is low on cortisol in the morning and has a difficult time arising and awakening, a small

(2.5mg) dose of IR hydrocortisone in a rapid dissolve tablet or sublingual troche can utilized. Patient should keep the dose bedside and take it 15-30 minutes before he or she needs to get out of bed, then continue with regular schedule of hydrocortisone for the remainder of the day.

Hydrocortisone dosing should be tapered over time. The goal is to obtain normal function of the adrenal gland, and removal of the hydrocortisone is required eventually for normal function. Dose can be gradually reduced after 30-60 days, over a 6-month period of time in general. Exceptions will be necessary for the individual patient based on the stressors present and ability to make lifestyle modifications.

Endocrine Hormones

Because of the multiple interactions between cortisol and the other endocrine hormones, levels should be measured and restoration therapy provided as needed for estrogen, progesterone, testosterone, and DHEA. Insulin resistance should be addressed if applicable. Thyroid function should be assessed and addressed. Note that in women who are deficient in both testosterone and DHEA, supplementation with DHEA can raise both levels in 2-3 months and therefore testosterone might not need to be supplemented unless there is a more urgent need to increase testosterone.

Sleep Enhancement

Obtaining adequate and restful sleep is especially important to clinical success in an adrenally challenged patient. Sleep is the most beneficial time for the adrenal glands to regain normal health and function. Individuals vary greatly in what works best for creating better sleep patterns, but listed are some recommendations that help a majority of patients.

Patients need to change their attitude towards sleep. Instead of thoughts during the evening of how tired they are and how they do not sleep well, they should imagine a good night's sleep and how much better they will feel following it.

Patients need to change the environment in which they sleep. Television sets and radios should be removed from the bedroom. All sources of lights should be removed. The bedroom should be used only for sleep (with the exception of romantic interactions).

Patients should go to bed early, even if they are not yet tired, by 9 or 10 p.m. in most cases. Obtain at least 8 hours of sleep, but more when possible. Sleep in on non-work days; allow the partner to be responsible for children or anything else that needs to be addressed in the morning.

Avoid prescription and OTC sleep aids. Avoid third shift work. Avoid excessive alcohol, especially close to bedtime. Avoid or reduce use of nicotine and caffeine.

Supplements that may help include theanine, 5HTP, PS, and magnesium as mentioned above. Theanine produces increased alpha brain wave activity inducing a relaxed, calm mental state. If theanine helps induce sleep but wears off during the night due to its short duration of action, it can be compounded into a slow release preparation.

Oral progesterone produces a significant amount of the metabolite 4-allo-pregnanolone which has GABA agonist activity or GABA itself can be supplemented to obtain anti-anxiety effects.

Adaptogens and or phosphatidylserine can be used to lower high cortisol levels that may be interfering with sleep. If a patient is awakening at night and brain is active, he/she may be experiencing hypoglycemia which is followed by a rise in cortisol. If this is the case, a small amount of protein consumed before bedtime can prevent the problem. A handful of almonds or a little protein on a piece of cracker (gluten-free recommended) will usually suffice.

High cortisol suppresses production of melatonin. Melatonin can be supplemented at a dose 0.5 to 1.5 mg oral or 0.25 to 0.5 mg sublingually 30 to 60 minutes before bedtime.

Additionally, relaxation and sleep induction may be helped by calming herbs including valerian root, chamomile, hops, and passion flower.

Lifestyle Modifications

The most challenging part of the process of recovery from adrenal dysfunction is also the most important and effective part of the process.....lifestyle modifications. Just as dealing satisfactorily with patient symptoms of hormone imbalance without addressing adrenal issues is nearly impossible, successfully dealing with adrenal issues without patient lifestyle adjustments is impossible. No combination of vitamins, minerals, adaptogens, sleep agents, and hormones will suffice to adequately treat symptoms without a significant change in the environment that created the situation.

- Stress reduction

    o Identify and eliminate or adjust stressful situations.

    o Say no to doing too much.

    o Do not feel guilty for taking care of yourself.

- Stress reaction adaptation: adjust attitude and physical response to stress.

    o Practice something that relaxes and helps to reduce stress *daily*. Schedule it and make it non-optional to enjoy yourself at least 10-15 minutes every day. Examples would be walking, bicycling, swimming, reading, yoga, meditation. Watching TV does not generally relax most people, depending on content.

    o Focus on the positive aspects of life to offset the stressors. Incorporate spirituality or religiosity. Include daily prayer and meditation. The Bible says it is not our place to worry. Let God (and your mother) do the worrying.

- Physical adjustments

    o Exercise regularly, at least 4 times a week. Gentle to mild exercise as tolerated. Do not exercise to the point of fatigue. Tai Chi, Yoga, Pilates, walking, swimming, etc.

    o Take breaks from work during the day. Lie down if possible.

- Get physical, emotional, and mental rest as much as possible.

- Laugh. Incorporate things into your daily life that make you laugh.

- Love. Meditate on it, express it, feel it.

Dietary Modifications

- Eat regular meals. Do not skip breakfast.

- Chew well.

- Take digestive enzymes before each meal.

- Eat good protein with each meal.

- Increase whole foods consumption.

    o Vegetables, nuts, beans, fruits (except bananas and melons)

- Decrease simple carbohydrate consumption.

- Avoid or limit alcohol intake.

- Avoid artificial sweeteners, flavorings, colorings, and preservatives.

- Avoid processed foods, hydrogenated fats, refined carbohydrates, animal fat, sodas, fruit juices, power drinks, caffeine, nicotine, and chocolate.

- Consume at least 1 teaspoonful of unrefined salt daily.

Example Adrenal Dysfunction Protocols

Note: all protocols include lifestyle recommendations above, as well as assessing status of sex steroids, thyroid, and insulin.

Cortisol levels are high throughout the day:
"Wired but tired feeling"

- Water: Ounces to consume daily should equal weight in pounds divided by 2.

- Unrefined salt: Consume as much as desired, but at least ½ teaspoonful twice a day.

- Adaptogens: Dose during day and at bedtime.

- PS in the evening to suppress bedtime cortisol. May give during the day also if adaptogens alone are not sufficient.

- Theanine 100-200 mg 2-4 times a day if anxious.

- Magnesium Glycinate 400-600 mg at bedtime.

- Vitamin/mineral support specific for the adrenals (along with daily MVM).

Cortisol elevated in the morning and at night but low or low-normal during the day:
"Wired, then tired, then restless"

- Water: Ounces to consume daily should equal weight in pounds divided by 2.

- Unrefined salt: Consume as much as desired, but at least ½ teaspoonful twice a day

- Adaptogens: Dose in morning and evening at least.

- PS in evening, no later than 6-7 pm.

  o Additional sleep agents p.r.n.

- Theanine 100-200 mg in late afternoon or evening and again before bedtime if anxious.

- Magnesium Glycinate 400-600 mg at bedtime.

- Vitamin/mineral support specific for the adrenals (along with daily MVM). Minimal dose of t.i.d.

- May consider adrenal glandular for low daytime cortisol levels if energy level is significantly low during the day and a more rapid recovery is desired.

- Check levels and restore DHEA and testosterone levels if low. May need to reduce dosage as adrenal health is addressed.

- Check progesterone levels and restore p.r.n. Use oral progesterone with sleep issues

Cortisol high in morning, but low the rest of the day
"Wired, then tired"

- Water: Ounces to consume daily should equal weight in pounds divided by 2.

- Unrefined salt: Consume as much as desired, but at least ½ teaspoonful twice a day.

- Adaptogens: at least at bedtime.

- Adrenal glandular at least t.i.d.

- Adrenal vitamin/mineral support at least t.i.d.

- Check levels and restore DHEA and testosterone levels if low. May need to reduce dosage as adrenal health is addressed.

- Check progesterone levels and restore p.r.n. Use oral progesterone with sleep issues.

- Natural insomnia agents, natural anti-anxiety agents p.r.n.

Cortisol below normal entire testing period
"Tired, just tired all the time"

- Water: Ounces to consume daily should equal weight in pounds divided by 2.

- Unrefined salt: consume as much as desired, but at least ½ teaspoonful twice a day.

- Adaptogens: at least at bedtime.

- Adrenal glandular at maximum recommended dose.

- Adrenal vitamin/mineral support at maximum recommended dose.

- Check levels and restore DHEA and testosterone levels if low. May need to reduce dosage as adrenal health is addressed.

- Check progesterone levels and restore p.r.n. Use oral progesterone with sleep issues.

- Hydrocortisone therapy as above.

- Insomnia agents, anti-anxiety agents p.r.n.

Caution: When using nutritional products that contain any combination of adrenal vitamins and minerals, adaptogens, phosphatidylserine, and glandular extracts, be sure the product provides therapeutic amounts of each of the ingredients.

Chapter Ten
A Functional Approach to Hypothyroidism

When symptoms of hypothyroidism exist in a patient, a comprehensive look at all the possible causes needs to be undertaken. These include:

- Autoimmune reactions affecting the thyroid gland

- Lack of production of the hormone from the gland

- Poor conversion of T4 to T3, decreased absorption of T3 into the cells

- Decreased intracellular transport of T3

- Less than optimal thyroid receptor function.

A functional approach requires determining the origin of the symptoms, and attempting to correct these issues in order to obtain optimal function of the thyroid gland, metabolism of the hormones, and hormone receptor response. Standard thyroid tests with a few additional nutritional tests can be used to determine which of the above issues are playing a role in an individual's symptoms. An attempt should be made to optimize function through nutritional and lifestyle changes before initiation of thyroid replacement therapy. In patients already taking thyroid replacement therapy but still experiencing symptoms, adjustments to therapy should be made in correlation with determination and correction of underlying causes.

Many of the conditions leading to less than optimal thyroid function involve lifestyle choices and nutrition. These include sex steroid hormone imbalances, adrenal issues, gut inflammation, poor blood sugar metabolism, chronic infections, and immune system dysfunction. Correcting causes can be challenging and most often takes time to accomplish. Correcting thyroid issues requires patience; long term functional resolution is not a quick process.

Autoimmune reactions are the number one cause of all thyroid disorders and, therefore, should be checked in every patient exhibiting significant symptoms of hyperthyroidism or hypothyroidism. Thyroid Peroxidase (TPO) antibody testing will reveal a thyroid autoimmune reaction the majority of the time.

Additional antibody testing, if desired, includes Thyroglobulin Antibody (TgAb) and Thyroid Stimulating Hormone Receptor Antibody (TRAb).

An autoimmune reaction in the thyroid gland destroys glandular cells and releases stored T4. This results in elevated peripheral T4 levels followed by elevated T3 levels due to conversion. Both suppress TSH, and levels of T4 and T3 then drop to below normal. A period of hyperthyroidism is followed by a more prolonged period of hypothyroidism. Subsequent attacks lead to more destruction of thyroid gland cells, lowering the ability to produce and store T4 and eventually to continual hypothyroidism (Hashimoto's).

Because it is impossible to assess at what stage the autoimmune reaction and attack is occurring, results of thyroid testing can be confusing. An autoimmune reaction involving the thyroid can skew the levels of TSH, T4, and T3, making interpretation difficult. Unless and until the autoimmune issue is addressed and controlled, long term satisfactory symptom resolution is difficult to achieve. (See Appendix G, "Approaches to Autoimmune Reactions".)

Production of thyroid hormone does not normally decline until age 50 to 55 years. Production is best measured by a Total T4 (TT4) level. If only Free T4 (fT4) level is measured and the result is lower than normal, this could be due to either low production or excessive binding, or a combination of both.

If the thyroid gland is producing less than an optimal amount of levothyroxine (T4), before thyroid therapy is initiated, determination of the reason for sub-optimal production should be investigated. Possible common causes include:

- Low substrates for T4

- Stress induced "sluggish" thyroid

- Pituitary hypofunction

- Poor nutrition

- Thyroid gland destruction

- Genetic defects

The main substrates for production of T4 are iodine and tyrosine. Iodine deficiency is a common problem and should be assessed and treated in all patients with low T4 production (See "Iodine Testing", Appendix H). Excess of the halogens bromide, fluoride and chloride can displace iodine and lead to a functional iodine deficiency. Tyrosine is not usually a problem, but there can be competition for absorption of amino acids, and low tyrosine has been noted in vegans and body builders.

Acute or chronic stress raises CRH and cortisol, both of which suppress TSH and lower production of thyroid hormones. Recovery does not always occur after a stressor has been eliminated, and thyroid production may remain sub-optimal. If patient history indicates a major stressor in the previous 6-18 months, sluggish thyroid caused by high cortisol should be considered a possibility even if cortisol values have returned to normal. Use of a thyroid glandular preparation may reestablish the ability of the thyroid gland to produce optimal amounts. The glandular product can be administered for a month or two and then withdrawn and levels checked. In some cases, production remains normal only as long as the patient remains on the glandular support.

In some cases of low thyroid hormone production, the thyroid gland is capable of producing adequate hormone, but is not receiving the signal to do so. Low TSH in this case can be caused by chronic stressors which fatigue the pituitary gland. Pregnancy and unnecessary or excessive Thyroid Replacement Therapy (ThRT) can also suppress TSH.

Support for low TSH includes addressing any adrenal dysfunction, use of a pituitary glandular, rubidium, L-arginine, and sage leaf. Vitamins and minerals that play a role in formation and release of TSH and the formation of thyroid hormone include pyridoxal-5-phosphate, riboflavin, niacin, magnesium, manganese, selenium, zinc, and copper. In addition to iodine and tyrosine, nutritional support for the formation of T4 includes ashwagandha, Vitamin A, Vitamin D, selenium, and zinc.

In conditions in which thyroid gland destruction occurs, low production of thyroid hormone cannot always be corrected by lifestyle modification and nutritional support alone. Sources of gland destruction include autoimmune thyroid reactions and heavy metal toxicities. If a significant amount of thyroid glandular cells have been destroyed, even removing or abating the cause of destruction will not allow T4 production to achieve optimal levels, and Thyroid Replacement Therapy (ThRT) will be required.

Functional hypothyroidism is a term used to describe the condition in which T4 levels are optimal but symptoms are present, due to excess binding and/or improper metabolism of the thyroid hormones resulting in a less than optimal amount of the active free T3 (fT3).

Excess binding caused by increased levels of Thyroid Binding Globulin (TBG) can be the result of administration of oral estrogens (including oral contraceptives), estrogen in excess of normal physiologic levels, pregnancy, administration of oral thyroid replacement, and chronic sleep disturbances. Both excess estrogen and thyroid can increase TBG, but it takes several months to reach the full effect. Therefore, retesting of thyroid levels should not be done within at least 90 days following any dosage change in either therapy. Testing 30 days after a change in thyroid therapy does not indicate the full net effect of the change on the amount of free hormone! Normally, very small amounts of thyroid hormone exist in the free or unbound state. Only 0.04% of the T4 present and 0.04% of the T3 present is unbound. Therefore, even small changes in TBG can have a significant effect on the amount of free hormone available to act on the thyroid receptors.

A common clinical scenario occurs when a patient temporarily feels better after being given thyroid hormone replacement therapy and a return to the practitioner in a few weeks shows some symptom response and normal thyroid levels. The administration of the hormone, or an increase in dosage, results in a temporary increased amount of the free hormone. However, the patient returns within the next few months with a return of symptoms. This is caused by the slow increase of TBG over the course of several months in response to the initiation or increase in oral thyroid therapy. Furthermore, if a patient is administered any T4 in their therapy and is converting to T3 poorly, therapy results in an increase in the disproportionate ratio of rT3 to T3, which can result in a worsening of symptoms.

Poor conversion of fT4 to the active fT3 is most likely the number one cause of Subclinical Hypothyroidism. Even if TSH is in a controlled study with ThRT, a number of studies have demonstrated Subclinical Hypothyroidism is associated with significant symptoms and increased risk for morbidity and mortality. Patients suffering from subclinical hypothyroidism can exhibit normal values for the production of thyroid hormones, but still experience symptoms of low thyroid function. Treatment is warranted despite normal TSH and TT4 levels, and consists of attempting to improve conversion of T4 as well as methods to increase function of the thyroid receptor.

Receptors specific to T4 have never been identified, and T4 should be viewed as a pro-hormone which is converted to the active hormone T3 in peripheral tissue. Approximately 80% of the T4 produced by the thyroid gland is converted peripherally to approximately equal amounts of T3 and reverse T3 (rT3). T3 is formed by the removal of an iodine molecule at the 5' position while reverse T3 is formed by iodine removal at the 5 position. rT3 is considered inactive by some references; however, it binds to the T3 receptor, has 1% of the activity of T3, and being an antagonist of T3, rT3 effectively blocks the action of T3 at the receptor level. The proper metabolism of T4 is therefore required to produce the proper balance or ratio of T3 and rT3. An excess of rT3 can block the metabolic effects of T3 even when T3 levels are optimal. *Whenever T4 therapy is administered, whether alone or in combination with T3 therapy, obtaining the desired metabolic effects of the T4 depends on proper conversion to T3.*

T4 is metabolized to T3 by the enzyme 5'deiodinase. Any factor that reduces the activity of this enzyme reduces conversion of T4 to T3, and conversion to reverse T3 (rT3) is proportionally increased. The same 5'deiodinase enzyme also converts rT3 to diiodothyronine (T2), so inhibition of the enzyme reduces clearance of rT3, resulting in a further increase in rT3 levels. Deiodination is also tissue-specific: type I deiodinase (D1), dependent on selenium and found primarily in the liver, kidneys, thyroid, and pituitary glands, produces 50% of the total plasma T3 and degrades rT3. The non-selenium-dependent type II deiodinase (D2) converts T4 to T3 locally in the central nervous system, pituitary, thyroid, skeletal muscle, and heart and also produces 50% of the circulating T3, while a third type, type III (D3) primarily inactivates T3 and T4 in the CNS. The various forms of the enzyme are affected by different factors; therefore TSH production in the pituitary stimulated by local T3 production does not necessarily reflect peripheral conversion in muscle and other tissue, which is why TSH levels can remain normal when symptoms reflect the improper conversion of T4 outside of the brain.

Factors that can inhibit the 5'deiodinase enzyme include*:

- Nutritional Deficiencies

  o Selenium, zinc, chromium, iodine

  o Vitamins A, B2, B6, B12, and E

  o Iron, copper

- Medications

  o Glucocorticoids, beta blockers, SSRIs, opiates, phenytoin, theophylline, lithium

  o Antibiotic use

  o Low progesterone

  o Chemotherapy

- Lifestyle and Environmental Issues

  o Stress (high cortisol)

  o Aging

  o Alcohol

  o Obesity

  o Cigarette smoking

  o Chronic inflammation or infection

  o Kidney disease and liver disease

- o Starvation

- o Mercury and lead

- o Growth Hormone Deficiency

- o Hemochromatosis

- o Pesticides

- o Radiation

- o Excessive soy, cruciferous vegetables, or α-Lipoic Acid

*Adapted from <u>Overcoming Thyroid Disorders</u> by David Brownstein, M.D.

Functional hypothyroidism therefore occurs when T4 metabolism produces an excess of rT3 in relation to T3. Treatment should consist of reducing high cortisol levels, removing sources of glucocorticoids, replacing nutritional factors affecting the 5'deiodinase enzymes that are deficient, and making lifestyle adjustments as needed. Reduction of the production of rT3 is critical, as when rT3 reaches high levels, it further inhibits the 5'deiodinase enzyme, especially in the liver.

Functional Hypometabolism

Symptoms of low thyroid function can persist when all thyroid levels are optimal, indicating good production, normal binding, and proper metabolism. The term "functional hypometabolism" refers to cases in which balancing the hormone levels at optimal levels does not produce the expected effects on metabolism. This situation has also been referred to as thyroid hormone resistance. In order to produce a metabolic effect, the fT3 must be absorbed into the cell, transported to the nucleus of the cell, bind with the T3 receptor, and receptors must be present in good quantity and be optimally functional.

Causes of functional hypometabolism include:

- Chronic high or low levels of cortisol

- Sub-optimal levels of Vitamin D

- Sub-optimal levels of ferritin

- Excess of progesterone

- Lack of PGC-1α activity

- Receptor dysfunction originating from toxicities

- Genetic disorders of the receptors

Thyroid receptor function is optimal when **cortisol** levels are normal. Persistently low and/or high cortisol levels will affect other areas of thyroid functions in addition to less responsive receptors. For example, high cortisol suppresses TSH and blocks the conversion of T4 to the active T3. Chronically low cortisol levels will reduce absorption into the cell and the number of thyroid receptors.

Jeffery Bland, PhD first reported several years ago at a meeting of the Institute for Functional Medicine that low **Vitamin D** levels can result in symptoms of hypothyroidism, and there are some supporting reports in the literature. Vitamin D levels need to be in the range of 50-70 ng/mL in order to obtain an optimal thyroid receptor response.

Iron deficiency, assessed by measuring serum **ferritin** (a more reliable measure of iron stores than serum iron levels) impairs thyroid hormone synthesis because of the dependence of thyroid peroxidase (TPO) activity on iron, and this can result in hypothyroidism. Ferritin also plays an important role in the transport of T3 within the cell to the nucleus. Ferritin levels need to be in the range of 90-110 for optimal thyroid function. Ferritin levels can be raised by administration of ferrous sulfate injections (very painful), or oral iron replacement therapy. Ferrous glycinate (iron glycinate) or an amino acid chelated iron supplement can raise the levels of ferritin with a much lower incidence of gastrointestinal disturbances than the traditional iron replacement products.

Functional hypometabolism can also theoretically result from excess amounts of essential fatty acids, Vitamin D, or progesterone, as first heard at a lecture by George Gillson, M.D., PhD. All three of these substances form a heterodimer with the retinoic acid receptor (RXR), as does T3. In theory, an excess of any of the four could cause excessive consumption of the RXR receptor, resulting in lower activity of the other three at the receptor level. Therefore, although a physiologic amount of progesterone enhances thyroid activity, excessive progesterone can cause functional hypometabolism.

PGC-1α is a transcription protein that has been found to be a key in the regulation of mitochondrial synthesis. PGC-1α also acts as a co-activator for neurotransmitter and hormone receptor sites, including T3, GABA, serotonin, and the sex steroids. T3 regulates PGC-1α through a T3 mediated expression of a thyroid hormone response element. At this point there is no commercial test available to measure levels of PGC-1α. Strategies to raise the level or activity of PGC-1α include:

- Increase cAMP

  o Exercise, α-Lipoic Acid

- Increase Nitric Oxide

    o Exercise, arginine, hawthorn & bloodroot, resveratrol

- Stimulate SIRT1 deacetylase (activates PGC-1α)

    o NAD

Optimal vs. Normal Levels

To determine normal reference ranges, a large number of people without symptoms of thyroid excess or deficiency are tested. The established normal ranges contain values at both ends of the tested ranges, which represent a very small number of individuals compared to the total number tested. If one were re-placing the level of hormone in a person who suddenly had all sources of endogenous hormone removed, the best odds of the patient having no symptoms would occur at the hormone level corresponding to the midpoint of the normal range. For example, if your thyroid gland were surgically removed, reestablishing your thyroid hormone level to the value corresponding to the midpoint of the normal range would give you the best chance of maximizing therapeutic outcome and not exhibiting symptoms. The chance of symp-toms occurring is minimized by not maintaining levels that would correlate with the values more towards either end of the curve. We should not allow patients that exhibit symptoms to remain at values that devi-ate too far from the midpoint of the normal range. A good strategy is to eliminate 25% from each end of the normal levels, and refer to the remaining range as the *optimal* level. Maintaining these optimal rather than "normal" levels in patients should result in a significant improvement in symptom management.

Thyroid Gradient Levels

The Thyroid Gradient Levels (TGL) is a tool that can be used to plot a patient's thyroid hormone levels relative to each other, and thus show where problems may be occurring that lead to the symptoms of hypothyroidism. Levels of total T4 (TT4), free T4 (fT4), and free T3 (fT3) are charted on the diagrams showing the patient's results within the reference range for each substance. Comparison of where the pa-tient's results are for one level in relationship to another can identify the degree of binding and conversion compared to normal. (See Appendix I for an explanation and example.)

Functional Thyroid Testing

Specific basic testing should be done on all patients that exhibit symptoms of hypothyroidism. Auto-immune issues should always be checked by including at least a TPO antibody test. Testing should allow for evaluation of production, binding, conversion, as well as include factors that affect thyroid absorption and transport, and thyroid receptor function, as explained below.

Low basal body temperature (BBT) indicates low metabolism, but it does not indicate the cause(s) of the symptoms. However, BBT measurement is an excellent tool for both practitioners and patients to track progress. BBT is recommended initially and at monthly intervals until symptom resolution is obtained.

Initial Basic Functional Thyroid Testing:

- TT4, fT4 (direct), fT3 (direct), TSH, TPO, Vitamin D, and ferritin with serum or dried capillary blood spot testing

- 4 point saliva cortisol

- Basal Body Temperature

Important note: patient should be at *complete* rest for *at least* 15 minutes prior to blood sample being taken

Initial Full Functional Thyroid Testing:

- All of the above and add iodine, and TgAb (if autoimmune issue strongly suspected)

Note: iodine testing – use urine testing. (See Appendix H on iodine testing)

- If symptoms of hormonal imbalance exist, measure E2, progesterone, testosterone, and DHEA (or DHEAS). Saliva or dried blood spot preferred methods.

Important note: Patient should be at *complete* rest for *at least* 15 minutes prior to blood sample being taken

Follow-up Testing:

Always do fT4, fT3, TSH, and TPO. Remainder of tests can be repeated as necessary depending on individual case

Interpretation of Test Results

- Basal Body Temp: ≥ one degree lower than normal on 3-day average indicates less than optimal metabolism

- TT4 is most accurate assessing thyroid hormone production

- Comparison of fT4 and TT4 provides assessment of binding (see "Thyroid Gradient Levels(T-GL)" explanation Appendix I)

- Comparison of fT3 and fT4 provides assessment of peripheral conversion of T4 to T3 (see TGL explanation Appendix I)

- Antibody testing should always be included as autoimmune issues are the number one cause of all thyroid problems. TPO will show reaction most often, but if an autoimmune issue is strongly suspected, may add TgAb also (see autoimmune strategies)

- Vitamin D is necessary for optimal thyroid receptor function. Vitamin D should be 60-80ng/mL for optimal thyroid receptor function

- Ferritin affects thyroid intracellular transport and utilization. Ferritin levels need to be 90-110ng/mL for optimal thyroid hormone transport and utilization

- Iodine affects thyroid production, metabolism, and receptor activity

- Abnormal cortisol levels affect thyroid function in multiple ways (See section on "Adrenal Dysfunction")

Reverse T3 (rT3) may also be measured if desired. Comparing rT3 to fT3 can also provide indication of conversion of T4 to T3 (See TGL explanation Appendix I). rT3 testing is not done by most labs, and is outsourced, commonly delaying reporting of results. This test involves the use of radioactive material, which makes it expensive and not earth friendly. Since interpretation of conversion can be accomplished by comparing fT3 to fT4, rT3 testing should be reserved for selected cases.

Thyroid panels that include "uptake" or "index" results should not be used. These results are not reliable to evaluate binding and metabolism of thyroid hormones. These values are not actual measurements; the uptake is an estimation of binding and the index is a calculated result based on the estimation. These tests are much less accurate and reliable than direct measurement of fT4 and fT3, but some labs continue to use and market them because the expense of producing a result is minimal so profit margins are greater.

Important note: Thyroid Binding Globulin levels can change with any change in thyroid (or estrogen) replacement therapy. Binding protein changes take place slowly and can occur over several months. **Re-testing should not be done for at least 90 days after any change in therapy to better ensure obtaining the net result on TBG and free hormones resulting from the change in therapy.**

Timing of testing sample vs. last dose of thyroid replacement therapy:

If patient is taking thyroid medication, the time of the last dose should be timed vs. the blood sampling to best represent the levels produced by the medication (avoiding peaks and troughs).

If patient is taking T4 alone (Synthroid, levothyroxine): testing sample should be obtained 4-16 hours after the last dose.

      (T4 peaks in 2-4 hours and lasts 18-20 hours in a Euthyroid patient.)

If patient is taking IR T3 only (Cytomel): testing sample should be obtained 2-4 hours after the last dose.

      (T3 peaks in 1-2 hours, and declines toward baseline 4-6 hours after dose.)

If patient is taking combination of IR T4 and T3 (Armour), testing sample should be obtained 4 hours after last dose

If patient is taking compounded SR T4 and/or T3, testing sample should be obtained 4-8 hours after last dose.

      (Compounded SR capsules peak in 1-2 hours, and tail off after 10 hours.)

If medication is not taken the morning of testing and it has been 24 hours or more since the last dose, resulting levels more represent endogenous production and not those produced by the medication.

Note: no matter which thyroid supplementation is administered, sampling 4 hours after the last dose is appropriate

Thyroid Replacement Therapy Options

Choosing a thyroid replacement therapy based on the individual patient's circumstances is essential to successful therapeutic outcomes. For example, unless a patient is adequately converting T4 to T3, then any therapy containing T4 will result in increased production of rT3 and functional hypometabolism. Also, any patient that is producing an optimal amount of T4 will respond to any T4 supplementation with an increase in TBG and decreased endogenous production. Selection of a thyroid replacement should be based on consideration of a patient's production and metabolism as well as receptor function. Functional issues should be addressed prior to initiation of therapy.

Levothyroxine Sodium (L-thyroxine, T4)

Products commercially available containing T4 include Synthroid, Levothyroid, Levoxy, Eltrosin, and various generics.

The administration of T4 only therapy as the standard thyroid replacement therapy is based on the assumption that T4 is converted to T3 within the body. Therefore any patient that has less than optimal conversion of T4 to T3 will not obtain the desired metabolic effects of T4 only therapy. TSH and T4 levels may respond adequately to therapy while symptoms remain an issue with the patient.

Degree of oral absorption from commercial T4 products has been shown to vary from 48% to 80%. Degree of absorption is dependent on the product formulation as well as the character of the intestinal contents, and individual patient reactions. Most commercial T4 products contain lactose, which has been shown to interfere with absorption of thyroid up to 40%, and may account for the variability in absorption.

Liothyronine Sodium (Tri-iodothyronine, T3)

Products commercially available containing T3 include Cytomel tablets and Triostat injection, and generics.

T3 commercial tablets are immediate release and available in only limited strengths (5, 25, and 50 mcg). They may contain lactose.

Thyroid Desiccated Powder USP

Products containing desiccated thyroid include Armour Thyroid, Thyroid Strong, Thyrar, S-P-T, and Thyroid USP from various manufacturers.

Desiccated thyroid powder (DTP) is obtained from pork thyroid glands. 1 Grain of DTP contains 38 mcg of T4, 9 mcg of T3. More than 99% of desiccated thyroid powder is pork thyroid gland which is not identified as to specific contents nor standardized beyond the content of T4, T3, and iodine.

DTP contains a standardized ratio of T4:T3 of 4.2:1. The normal ratio of T4:T3 in the human body is approximately 3.3:1. Use of a standardized ratio of T4 and T3 would be appropriate only if the population using it were all converting at similar degrees of normal. A fixed ratio does not allow for individual changes in metabolism, or changes in metabolism over time within an individual. The patient optimally converting T4 to T3 will react better to DTP than a patient who has less than optimal conversion. Before DTP therapy is chosen for a patient, conversion should be evaluated and addressed.

DTP also contains T2, T1, selenium and calcitonin, which affect thyroid function. T2 and T1 may provide biological activity, but overall contribution is considered minimal. The amounts of these agents are not identified, quantified, or standardized. Therefore, when DTP is administered, agents which affect the function of the gland and system that is being treated are being provided in unknown and possibly inconsistent amounts.

The USP monograph for Desiccated Thyroid Powder includes the statement that it "may contain lactose, sucrose, dextrose, starch, or other suitable diluents". The suitable diluents used are not usually identified on the label. Caution should be taken as some of these diluents may not be suitable in individual patients. Additionally, lactose should not be considered a suitable diluent as lactose has been shown to interfere with thyroid absorption by as much as 40%.

Liotrix

Commercial products include Thyrolar and Euthroid tablets.

Liotrix is a mixture of synthetic T4 and T3 in a 4 to 1 ratio by weight in an immediate release tablet. Manufacturers differ on approximate equivalent strengths to desiccated thyroid powder.

Compounded Thyroid Preparations

Compounding pharmacies can prepare any combination of T3 and/or T4 in any strength, in both immediate release and slow release capsules. Compounders can also provide compounded desiccated thyroid powder preparations in non-commercially available strengths or in the case of unavailability of commercial products. With the advantages of combining therapies, providing slow release preparations, and adding adjunctive therapies, compounding may help improve patient compliance.

Synthetic vs. Natural

Use of the term synthetic or natural to describe thyroid replacement products is not appropriate. The terms were originally used for marketing purposes. Companies providing pork-sourced products used the term synthetic for the commercially available T3 and T4 products since they were made in a lab. The term natural was used for pork- sourced products because something "natural" has better overall acceptance with patients than something that is "synthetic".

Use of the term "natural" to describe products containing desiccated thyroid powder is not appropriate as it is not known how much of the pork product is natural to the human body. The bioidentical or natural T4 and T3 in desiccated pork thyroid only constitute less than 1% of the total powder. More than 99% of the powder is unidentified pork thyroid gland substance which may or may not be bioidentical or "natural" for humans.

Physiologic Bioidentical Thyroid Restoration Therapy

The important issues in thyroid replacement product options are whether the agent being administered is bioidentical to what a human produces, and whether it is being administered in a physiological manner. The T3 and T4 in all commercial and compounded preparations are all bioidentical to the human thyroid hormones. The differences, and therefore factors for appropriate product selection, are the other constituents of the products, the manner in which the hormone is delivered (immediate or slow release), and the ratio of T4 to T3 in combination products.

Maintaining normal physiologic levels with thyroid replacement is critical to long term success for symptom management correlated with optimal levels. Human production of T4 is approximately 100 mcg daily. Daily production of T3 is approximately 30 -35 mcg. If a patient had a thyroid gland removed or completely destroyed, a good physiologic dose of thyroid replacement would be 100 mcg of T4 with 30 mcg of T3. In most cases, thyroid replacement therapy is supplementing endogenous production to restore the levels to optimal. Therapy should be restoration therapy, designed to add to the endogenous production to bring the level back to an optimal level. Small amounts of thyroid hormones should be administered, starting at a low dose and increasing slowly as needed. Any dose seen by the brain as an excess to what would restore normal physiologic levels can result in increased binding, decreased endogenous production, and possibly decreased receptor response.

If TT4 levels are less than optimal, the first step in a functional approach should be to try to determine the cause of low production and correct the underlying cause. Before T4 therapy is initiated, conversion of T4 to T3 should be optimized. If T4 therapy is initiated, it should be dosed starting at 5 mcg to 10 mcg daily. With normal production of T4 being 100 mcg daily, it does not make sense physiologically to initiate replacement dosing at 50 mcg or 100 mcg daily. Even 25 mcg daily can be excessive in many individuals. Dosage can be increased if test results indicate a need, but retesting should not be done for at least 90 days after any therapy change to allow for net effect of any changes in TBG.

Before initiating T3 therapy, an attempt to optimize endogenous fT3 levels should be done by evaluation and treatment of any binding or conversion issues. If T3 therapy is initiated, it should be done at 2.5 mcg of T3 in a slow release preparation. The literature is clear that T3 would be the thyroid therapy of choice except for two problems with commercially available T3: it is available only in limited strengths and only in immediate release capsules. Both of these deficiencies in commercially available T3 can be overcome by using a compounded slow release T3 preparation.

T4 therapy does not require a slow release preparation. It can be compounded in a slow release preparation, which is often done to combine with T3 for improved compliance and decreased costs. An important factor to consider in the use of slow release products is the intestinal health of the individual patient.

If the gut is inflamed, there appears to be interference with the breakdown of the hydroxypropylmethyl-cellulose used to make slow release products. In cases where there may be significant gut inflammation (autoimmune diseases), then it is best to avoid the use of slow release products until the gut inflammation has been addressed. If T3 therapy needs to be dosed in an immediate release preparation because of gut issues, then it should be dosed at three times a day.

Whether to initially use a commercial product or a compounded thyroid preparation requires individual professional judgment. No matter which THRT product is used, metabolism and functional issues must be adequately addressed to obtain good therapeutic results. Many patients do not obtain adequate symptom relief on T4 therapy alone, but this could be due to the lack of addressing the functional thyroid issues and/or problems with inert ingredients. Some patients do well on desiccated thyroid USP products, at least for a significant period of time. But the active and inactive components of the pork-sourced product may cause issues in some patients, or the ratio of T4 to T3 may not be appropriate. Compounded preparations offer the advantages of pure bioidentical T4 and T3, in whatever strength and ratio is appropriate for each patient, and as immediate or slow release preparations.

Summary of Assessment and Treatment

For a patient presenting with hypothyroid symptoms (not on THRT):

- Have thyroid health evaluation form (Appendix E) completed

- Order thyroid tests

  o Initial basic functional tests: TT4, fT4 (direct), fT3 (direct), TSH, TPO, Vitamin D, and ferritin with serum or dried capillary blood spot testing, 4 point saliva cortisol

  o Have patient do basal body temperature testing (Appendix F)

     Or

  o **Initial Full Functional Thyroid Testing:**

     ▪ All of the initial basic tests plus add iodine, and TgAb (if autoimmune issue strongly suspected)

     ▪ Note: Iodine testing – use urine testing. See Appendix G on iodine testing.

     ▪ If symptoms of hormonal imbalance exist, measure E2, progesterone, testosterone, and DHEA (or DHEAS). Saliva or dried blood spot preferred methods.

Address any sex steroid imbalances, cortisol issues, and insulin resistance as determined by health questionnaires and testing.

If TPO or other antibody tests are positive (higher than normal):

- Address autoimmune issues as first priority. Note: Other thyroid levels may be skewed (Appendix G)

If TT4 is less than optimal:

- Check iodine level if not already done or trail therapy of low dose iodine (Appendix H)

- Check diet for tyrosine consumption and supplement if in doubt

- Stress issues producing a "sluggish thyroid": give thyroid glandular extract (or combination glandular extract that includes thyroid, pituitary, and adrenal extracts)

- Daily MVM plus additional B Complex, magnesium, selenium, and zinc

    o MVM may be tried initially with others added later if not successful in raising TT4

- If not successful in raising TT4 with lifestyle and nutritional functional factors in 2-3 months, restoration therapy can be initiated

If TT4 is optimal, but fT4 is less than optimal:

- Review causes of excessive binding and address as necessary

If fT3 is low in comparison to fT4:

- Review causes of poor conversion and address as necessary, especially stress and cortisol

- Basic supplementation includes daily MVM, selenium to a total of 400 mcg daily, zinc to a total of 50 mg daily and, if diabetic, chromium at 1000mcg daily.

If fT3 is high relative to fT4:

- Suspect autoimmune issue and address

- Was patient at complete rest for at least 15 minutes prior to sampling?

- Test iodine if not already done and supplement as needed (Appendix G)

If addressing functional issues does not resolve low thyroid levels in 2-3 months, restoration therapy can be initiated.

For patients already on thyroid therapy but with symptoms of hypothyroidism:

- Do thyroid level testing with appropriate timing relative to last dose of therapy.

  - See timing of testing sample vs. last dose of thyroid replacement therapy in section on Functional Thyroid Testing. If in doubt, draw sample 4 hours after the last dose

- If not already done, test cortisol and sex steroids and address

- Evaluate and address binding and conversion issues

- Test Vitamin D, ferritin, and iodine and correct as needed

- Daily MVM

- Treatment changes based on test results

  - Often dosages of THRT need to be reduced to physiological amounts. Decreasing dosage should not be done quickly as patients will feel worse. Decrease THRT dosage by no more than 25% at one time, and retest in no sooner than 90 days. Decreasing supraphysiologic doses may require a significant period of time.

  - T4 therapy may need decreasing while T3 therapy may require an increase. Use low doses (2.5-15 mcg) of T3 while slowly reducing T4 therapy.

The Functional Thyroid Approach in a Nutshell:

Address factors affecting the function of the thyroid gland and hormones: lifestyle, nutritional, and environmental.

Always address autoimmune issues firsthand.

Address sex steroids and cortisol issues.

Initiate thyroid restoration therapy after above have been addressed and are insufficient.

Be patient.

Chapter Eleven
Insulin Resistance

The most common and basic trigger of hormonal imbalance is insulin resistance. Excessive intake of refined flour, sugar, refined carbohydrates, saturated fat, and trans-hydrogenated fat contributes to rapid rise and fall of insulin levels, which leads to overproduction of cortisol. Elevated cortisol in turn interferes with the functions of estrogen, progesterone, and the function and production of testosterone. Chronic high cortisol eventually leads to increased progesterone conversion to cortisol, resulting in a state of relative estrogen dominance. Therefore, the cause of a woman exhibiting the symptoms of early menopause may be the development of insulin resistance, or elevated cortisol, or often a combination of both. Diet can be the most basic link between hormone imbalance and dysfunction.

Excessive intake of carbohydrates that are rapidly absorbed and subsequent obesity have been associated with increased risk of cancer, including breast cancer. Women who are overweight, especially those with abdominal fat, are more likely to suffer from hot flashes during the menopausal transition.

Establishing a healthy manner of eating is essential for functional hormone balance. Included in this concept would be:

- A low glycemic index diet for all patients who have developed or may be developing insulin resistance that most likely is at least contributing to their hormonal symptoms
- Eating small amounts of low glycemic index foods every 3-4 hours to keep blood sugar levels stable
- Consuming small amounts of healthy fats with carbohydrates to slow conversion to blood sugar
  - Healthy fats include those from fish, olive oil, flaxseed, nuts, etc.
  - Saturated fats in meat and dairy need to be eaten in moderation
  - Partially hydrogenated and trans fats need to be avoided
- Avoiding artificial sweeteners, high fructose corn syrup and its relatives
- Avoiding meat and dairy products that may have added hormones
- Including lean protein with every meal
- Avoiding all sweetened drinks – soda, fruit juices, sports or energy drinks

Attaining and maintaining symptom management with hormonal balance must include addressing insulin resistance. Otherwise you will be fighting an uphill, lifelong, unwinnable battle.

Chapter Twelve
Functional Hormone Balance

A functional approach to hormone balance requires assessing and addressing the underlying causes of the symptoms or issues. Hormone supplementation is part of the functional approach when hormone levels are deficient due to the natural process of aging. However, whenever a hormone level is low for the specific age of the patient and not typical for that age, the question should always be asked, what caused the lower than normal level?.

For example, a female, age 25, presents with symptoms of PMS or PCOS, and her test results show low progesterone. Progesterone supplementation, inositol, and natural anti-inflammatory agents in addition to an anti-inflammatory diet should be considered for this patient. However, many times the low progesterone is caused by irregular ovulation, which is caused by FHS/LH imbalances, which is caused by developing insulin resistance, which is caused by a combination of poor diet, inadequate exercise, and improper sleep habits. If these underlying lifestyle issues are not addressed and corrected, then the causes of the problems are not being addressed. If the lifestyle issues are not corrected, then most likely there will be additional hormonal imbalance issues in the coming years even if the above suggestions address the present symptoms.

The same issue can occur with male patients. If a male patient, age 42, has a testosterone level of a 70-year-old, the question should be asked why his level is so low. Often with males, a lack of exercise, obesity, stress, and poor sleep habits can decrease natural testosterone production. Aromatase enzyme, which converts testosterone to estrogen, is produced and stored in adipose tissue. Cortisol increases aromatase activity. The overweight patient with stress produces high estrogen, which suppresses LH and therefore testosterone production. Less testosterone is produced, and a greater percentage of what is produced is converted to estrogen. This patient would benefit from testosterone supplementation for symptom management, but he may convert much of the supplemented testosterone to estrogen, creating more issues. If the underlying lifestyle issues are not addressed, he will have future hormone issues, and the underlying causes of his symptoms are not being addressed.

In both of these examples, hormone supplementation without addressing the functional cause of the symptoms is using hormones in a way similar to the manner in which most drugs are used. The hormone is being used to treat the symptoms, not the cause of the symptoms. In most cases such as these, symptom management is not maintained long term, and, often, supplementation in excess of physiologic amounts may be needed to control symptoms long term. At higher doses, all the protective benefits of the hormones are not necessarily maintained.

In a functional approach to hormone balance, addressing the lifestyle issues such as diet, sleep, and exercise is critical to long term success of restoration therapy. Because so many vitamins and minerals are important as co-factors in enzymatic reactions involving conversion, metabolism, and receptor functions for the hormones, every patient should be supplemented with a trustworthy daily MVM. Proper liver function is also essential to optimal function of the hormones. Liver detoxification should be considered in most patients if there is any history of exposure to environmental toxins, xenoestrogens, and/or poor diet.

In summary, functional physiologic hormone restoration therapy is not just replacing deficient hormones. Consideration of underlying issues leading to hormone deficiencies and imbalances are also assessed, including:

- Diet

- Nutrition

- Sleep habits

- Exercise

- Stress

- Weight management

- Environmental influences

- Liver function

- Inflammation

- Infections, including yeast

Nothing leads to better long term management of "hormonal" symptoms in patients than creating an environment where balanced physiologic levels of hormones can function optimally.

Selected References and Resources

Textbooks

Seifer D.B., Speroff L., Clinical Gynecologic Endocrinology and Infertility, 7th Edition 2004 *Lippincott Williams & Wilkins (LWW)*

The Use of Estrogens and Progestogens in Clinical Practice Edited By Fraser I. , Jansen R., Lobo R. , Whitehead M. , Jan 1999 Churchill Livingstone

Nutritional Medicine, Alan R. Gaby, MD, 2011, Fritz Perlberg Publishing, Concord, NH

Testosterone: Action•Deficiency•Substitution, Edited by Eberhard Nieschlag and Hermann M. Behre, 3rd Edition, 2004, Cambridge University Press, United Kingdom

Werner & Ingbar's The Thyroid: A Fundamental and Clinical Text, 9th Edition, 2005, Lippincott Williams & Wilkins, Philadelphia, PA

Textbook of Nutritional Medicine, Melvyn R. Werbach, 1999, Third Line Press Inc., Tarzana, CA

Textbook of Functional Medicine, David S. Jones, MD Editor in Chief, 2005 The Institute for Functional Medicine Gig Harbor, WA

Books

Hormone Harmony. Alicia Stanton MD and Vera Tweed. 2009. Healthy Life Library, Los Angeles, CA

What You Must Know About Women's Hormones. Pamela Wartian Smith, MD, MPH. 2010. Square One Publishers, Garden City Park, NY

You've Hit Menopause, Now What? 3 Simple Steps to Restoring Hormone Balance. George Gillson, MD, PhD and Tracy Marsden BScPharm. 2003. Blitzprint, Calgary, AB

Are Your Hormones Making You Sick?: A Woman's Guide to Better Health Through Hormonal Balance. Eldred B. Taylor, MD and Ava Bell Taylor, MD. 2003. Published by Physicians Natural

Medicine Inc, United States

Bioidentical Hormones 101. Jeffrey Dach, MD. 2011. iUniverse, Bloomington, IN

Awakening Athena: Resilience, Restoration, and Rejuvenation for Women. Kenna Stephenson, MD. 2004 Published by Health, Heart and Mind Institute, Tyler, Texas

What Your Doctor May Not Tell You About Breast Cancer: How Hormone Balance Can Help Save Your Life. John R. Lee, MD, David Zava PhD, and Virginia Hopkins. 2002. Warner Books, Inc., New York, NY

The Testosterone Syndrome. Eugene Shippen, MD. & William Fryer. 1998, M. Evans and Company Inc., New York, NY

Adrenal Fatigue: The 21st Century Stress Syndrome, James L. Wilson, ND, DC, PhD. 2001 Smart Publications, Petaluma, CA

Overcoming Thyroid Disorders. David Brownstein, MD. 2nd edition, 2008, Medical Alternative Press, West Bloomfield, MI

Why Do I Still Have Thyroid Symptoms When My Lab Tests Are Normal? Datis Kharrazian, DHSc, DC, MS. 2010, Morgan James Publishing, Garden City, NY

Literature

Holtorf K. The bioidentical hormone debate: are bioidentical hormones (estradiol, estriol, and progesterone) safer or more efficacious than commonly used synthetic versions in hormone replacement therapy? *Postgrad Med.* 2009 Jan;121(1):73-85. doi: 10.3810/pgm.2009.01.1949. Review. PMID:19179815

Schwartz E.T., Holtorf K. Hormones in Wellness and Disease Prevention: Common Practices, Current State of the Evidence, and Questions for the Future. *Prim Care Clin Office Pract* 35 (2008) 669–705

Stephenson K, Neuenschwander P.F., Kurdowska A.K. The effects of compounded bioidentical transdermal hormone therapy on hemostatic, inflammatory, immune factors; cardiovascular biomarkers; quality-of-life measures; and health outcomes in perimenopausal and postmenopausal women. *Int J Pharm Compd.* 2013 Jan-Feb;17(1):74-85. PMID:23627249

Joanna Y. Du, MD, Puy Sanchez, MD, Lila Kim, BS, Colleen G. Azen, MS, David T. Zava, PhD, and Frank Z. Stanczyk, PhD.

Percutaneous progesterone delivery via cream or gel application in postmenopausal women: a randomized cross-over study of progesterone levels in serum, whole blood, saliva, and capillary blood. *Menopause* 2013. Vol. 20, No. 11.

Stanczyk F.Z., Paulson R.J., Roy S. Percutaneous administration of progesterone: blood levels and endometrial protection. *Menopause.* 2005 Mar;12(2):232-7. Review. PMID:15772572

Du J.Y. , Sanchez P. , Kim L. , Azen C.G. , Zava D.T. , Stanczyk F.Z. . Percutaneous progesterone delivery via cream or gel application in postmenopausal women: a randomized cross-over study of progesterone levels in serum, whole blood, saliva, and capillary blood. *Menopause.* 2013 May 6. [Epub ahead of print]

Cavalieri E.L., Rogan E.G. Depurinating estrogen-DNA adducts in the etiology and prevention of breast and other human cancers. *Future Oncol* 2010;6(1):75-79.

E.L. Cavalieri, E.G. Rogan and D. Chakravarti. Initiation of cancer and other diseases by catechol ortho-quinones: A unifying mechanism. *CMLS* 2002; 59: 665-681

Websites

www.endotext.com

www.rain-tree.com

www.adrenalfatigue.org

www.ProactiveBreastWellness.com

Testing Labs

ZRT Laboratory   www.zrtlab.com

Appendix A
Basic BHRT Protocol

Balanced hormone restoration requires assessment and correlation of the patient's relevant medical history, symptoms, and hormone levels.

- Obtain medical history and note individual goals and pertinent history.

    o Have patient fill out the **Hormone Evaluation and Medical History** form (Appendix B)

- Obtain appropriate baseline testing of hormone levels

    o See "Appropriate Hormone Testing"

- Correlate patient symptoms with hormone levels to determine individual patient hormone needs

    o Symptoms -- See "Assessment of Hormonal Needs"

    o Key points

        ▪ Symptoms often classified as hormonal symptoms can be caused or aggravated by deficiency or excess individual sex steroids, cortisol, thyroid, insulin resistance, and nutritional deficiencies

        ▪ Symptoms of excessive hormone often mimic symptoms of deficiency of that hormone due to tachyphylaxis of the hormone receptor

        ▪ In the case of progesterone, excess can mimic the symptoms of estrogen deficiency as too much progesterone down-regulates estrogen receptors

        ▪ All possible causes of a symptom or set of symptoms should be investigated and addressed as needed

    o Restore hormone levels to physiologic levels of a 30-35 year old

        ▪ See section on **"Physiologic Dosing of Hormones"** and **"Dosing Guidelines"** (Appendix D)

        ▪ Key Points

- Hormone therapy is effective by a number of administration routes, including transdermal, oral, sublingual or buccal, injections, and subcutaneous pellets

- Choice of dosage route is based on the hormone(s) involved, pharmacokinetics, and individual patient preference

- Hormones should be initiated at the low end of the standard range and increased slowly

- Proper testing should be used to monitor levels, and appropriate type of testing depends on route of administration

    o See **"Appropriate Hormone Testing"**, Section 3

    o Recommend any necessary lifestyle recommendations

        ▪ Address patient dietary and nutritional intake

        ▪ Address sleep and exercise habits

- Monitor symptoms and re-test levels in 3-4 months

    o Adjust dosage as needed

    o Make lifestyle adjustments as needed

- Monitor levels and symptom changes at least once a year for first 2 years of therapy

Hormone Testing Considerations

- Appropriate baseline testing should be performed.

- Pre-menopausal or peri-menopausal women should test on days 18-21 of cycle. All other patients can test on any day. If cortisol testing is included, test should be done on a day of "average stress".

- Serum testing can be used for baseline testing with the following considerations kept in mind:

    o Normal ranges for estrogens and progesterone are wide and many patients can begin to exhibit symptoms while still within the low normal or high normal ranges.

    o Most labs still use the same androgen testing procedures that were developed for measuring in males, and these are not sensitive enough for women. Most labs report one normal range for DHEA and testosterone for all adult women regardless of age. This is due to the fact that the test is not sensitive enough to give ranges per age group, so the result is not useful clinically. Testing androgens in women with most serum labs is a total waste of the patient's time and money.

o Serum testing is not valid for administration of topical hormones. Although used and suggested by many, it has never been validated for such. Validation would require either direct comparison to tissue levels and/or correlation to long term overall effects, neither of which has been done. Frank Stanczyk's review article on topical progesterone proves that the tissue level in the uterus *does not* correlate with serum levels for topically applied progesterone.

o Serum testing with oral supplementation may result in higher levels than tissue, as the test result may include some metabolites. For example, Nahoul showed that the measurement for progesterone given orally included some of the major metabolites as well as progesterone.

o Serum testing measures total (bound and unbound) hormone in most cases and binding globulins, which can vary significantly, must be taken into consideration.

- Urine testing

  o Urine testing measures metabolites, not the hormones themselves, and is not necessarily reflective of the amount of hormone present in the tissue. When hormones are supplemented, urine testing does not reflect tissue levels. For example, if patient #1 is taking 100mg of oral progesterone, her 24-hour urine collection will show the metabolites for 100mg of progesterone, while less than 10% is available to the tissue as progesterone. If patient #2 applies 10 mg of progesterone topically, her 24-hour urine collection will reflect the metabolites of 10mg of progesterone. Comparing the results of the two patients, patient #1 will appear to have 10 times more progesterone in her system, although the topical administration of the 10mg of progesterone in patient #2 would result in tissue levels at least as high if not higher than patient #1.

  o Urine testing can be useful in determining how a patient is metabolizing his or her hormones, either endogenous or supplemented. This is discussed further in the section on "Safe Estrogen Metabolism".

- Saliva testing

  o Saliva testing, if done correctly, has been shown to correlate well with tissue levels of hormones. The most experienced and well-referenced saliva testing lab is ZRT Laboratory, as they are the only lab to correlate ten years' worth of patient data with levels. The observed or expected target range for each hormone is correlated with dosage, dosage route, and time of administration of the last dose as well as symptom management.

o Saliva testing is the only accurate method to obtain cortisol levels at 4 points throughout the day, which is necessary for proper adrenal assessment.

o Saliva testing cannot be used if any hormone is being administered by sublingual or buccal route. These routes of administration result in accumulation of hormone in the oral mucous membranes and tissues, resulting in a high level which does not correspond to tissue levels.

o Saliva testing should not be used if there is any oral bleeding present

o Saliva testing cannot be used to measure large proteins, such as thyroid hormones, PSA, LH, FSH, SHBG, etc.

o Caution must be taken with saliva testing not to contaminate the sample with fingers when topical hormones are used, or with any medications, lotions, or creams applied to the face.

- Capillary Blood Spot Testing (dried blood spot)

    o If patient is using topical hormones, contact with the fingers can result in higher levels than normal in the fingertips for several days. Caution must be taken not to contaminate the sample. Hands should never be used to apply a topical hormone.

- Combination testing

    o Some labs may offer a combination test kit, which includes both saliva and blood spot testing. This can be advantageous for obtaining cortisol results with saliva testing, thyroid results with capillary blood spot testing, and the sex steroids with either modality.

- Hormones to be tested

    o For females, always test estradiol (E2), progesterone, DHEA or DHEA Sulfate, testosterone, and cortisol 4 times in one day. These can all be measured in saliva, or the sex steroids in capillary blood spot and cortisol in saliva.

    ▪ Estradiol is adequate for baseline testing for estrogen status. Because estriol (E3) affects the function of E2, once estrogen supplementation is initiated, it is recommended to add estriol (E3) to the follow up testing to make sure both E2 and E3 are at physiologic levels.

- It is rare to find a peri-menopausal woman who does not have some degree of adrenal dysfunction, so cortisol testing is recommended as part of baseline testing.

- Thyroid testing should be done if symptoms of hypothyroidism exist (see thyroid protocol).

o For males, baseline testing should include estradiol, testosterone, DHEA or DHEA Sulfate, PSA, SHBG, and cortisol 4 times a day. Thyroid testing should be done if symptoms of hypothyroidism exist (see thyroid protocol). Baseline hematocrit is recommended prior to any testosterone supplementation.

- Follow-up testing should be done approximately 3 months following initiation of therapy

o May vary with individual but in general need to assure patient is not at higher than physiologic levels, even if patient's symptoms have been adequately addressed.

Symptoms Assessment Considerations

- Symptoms often classified as hormonal symptoms can be caused or aggravated by deficiency or excess individual sex steroids, cortisol, thyroid, insulin resistance, and nutritional deficiencies.

o Lack of physiological amounts of progesterone can appear as estrogen dominance and/or deficiency of estrogen. Progesterone at physiologic amounts is required for proper function of estrogen receptors. Progesterone stimulates production of estrogen receptors, but can also down-regulate estrogen receptor sensitivity in presence of excessive estrogen. Low progesterone therefore can mimic symptoms often thought of as related to low estrogen.

o Low progesterone also increases conversion of testosterone to DHT, causing symptoms commonly referred to as excessive testosterone (acne, oily skin, hair loss)

o High cortisol can block progesterone receptors, suppress testosterone production and function of testosterone receptors, and interfere with estrogen receptor function. High cortisol can also cause hypothyroidism by suppressing TSH, blocking conversion of T4 to the active T3, and decreasing function of the thyroid receptor. High cortisol also increases insulin resistance. *High cortisol therefore mimics symptomology of deficiency states of most other sex steroids as well as hypothyroidism and insulin resistance.*

o Chronic low cortisol results in decreased production of all steroid receptors, can increase conversion of progesterone to cortisol resulting in low progesterone levels, and decreased absorption of steroids into the cells. *Low cortisol therefore can mimic symptomology of deficiencies in all sex steroids, hypothyroidism, and insulin resistance.*

o Symptoms of low testosterone, low thyroid function, and poor nutrition overlap significantly. Patients with symptoms of low testosterone should be screened for low thyroid function (see thyroid protocol) and have their nutritional status assessed.

o Insulin resistance causes fluctuations in cortisol levels, leading to the problems described for high and low cortisol.

• Symptoms of excessive hormone often mimic symptoms of deficiency of that hormone due to tachyphylaxis of the hormone receptor.

o Hormones given in excess usually result in good initial response, as most hormones will up-regulate their own receptors temporarily as they are increased. After a period of time, the excess hormone results in tachyphylaxis, or down-regulation of hormone receptors and a return to the symptoms of hormone deficiency.

▪ Excessive estrogen down-regulates estrogen receptors resulting in symptoms of estrogen deficiency even though estrogen levels are high.

▪ Excessive testosterone down-regulates testosterone receptors resulting in symptoms of testosterone deficiency even though testosterone levels are high.

▪ In the case of progesterone, excess can mimic the symptoms of estrogen deficiency as too much progesterone down-regulates estrogen receptors.

o Time to tachyphylaxis will vary with the individual and the amount of excess, and the individual hormone, but in general:

▪ Excess estrogen will result in down-regulation of receptors in 1-2 months in females.

▪ Excess testosterone will result in down-regulation of receptors in 3-4 months in females.

▪ Excess testosterone in males results in down-regulation of receptors in 3-12 months.

- Excess progesterone in females will result in down-regulation of estrogen receptors in 2-6 months.

- All possible causes of a symptom or set of symptoms should be investigated and addressed as needed

    - When symptoms of a hormone deficiency are not adequately addressed with normal supplemental dosing and normal physiologic levels, other causes of the symptoms need to be thoroughly assessed. For example, for a patient receiving a normal dose of estrogen and maintaining a normal physiologic level that would control estrogen deficiency symptoms in the majority of women, if she is still experiencing hot flashes, then insulin resistance, cortisol output, hypothyroidism, and estrogen metabolism should be examined more closely before increasing the dose of estrogen.

- See "Symptom Lists" (Appendix C)

Confidential Hormone Evaluation/Medical History

Name:_____

Today's Date:_____ Birthdate: _____ Age: _____

Address: _____

City:_____ State:_____ Zip: _____

Phone: _____ E-mail Address: _____

Gender: □ Male   □ Female   Height: _____   Weight:_____

Current Physicians/Health Care Practitioners

Name, address, phone and email address (if known)

_____

_____

_____

_____

_____

Doctor Medical Release Authorization

"I hereby authorize my physician or health care provider to furnish an agent of _____ _____ any and all records pertaining to my medical history, services rendered, and/or treatments. I understand that employees of _____ will protect my privacy and this information will be released to other health care professionals only when necessary in order to provide health care services to me. I further understand that a _____ employee will not release this information unless authorized by me in writing."

Signature_____ Date: _____

Medical History

Medical Conditions/Diseases: Please check all that apply to you:

_____ Heart Disease (ex: Congestive Heart Disease)   _____ Blood Clotting Problems

_____ High Cholesterol or Lipids (ex: Hyperlipidemia)   _____ Diabetes or Insulin Resistance

_____ High Blood Pressure (Hypertension)   _____ Arthritis or Joint problems

_____ Fibromyalgia or Chronic Fatigue   _____ Depression

_____ Ulcers (stomach, esophagus)   _____ Epilepsy

_____ Thyroid Disease   _____ Headaches/Migraines

_____ Hormonal Related Issues   _____ Eye Disease

_____ Lung Condition (example: asthma, emphysema, COPD)

_____ Autoimmune Disease   If checked, type: _____

_____ Chronic Pain   If checked, type of pain: _____

_____ Cancer   If checked, type of cancer: _____

Other: Please list: _____

Patient name (please print): _____

Do you have a family history of any of the following?

Uterine Cancer	_____	Family member(s) _____
Ovarian Cancer	_____	Family member(s) _____
Breast Cancer	_____	Family member(s) _____
Fibrocystic Breast	_____	Family member(s) _____
Heart Disease	_____	Family member(s) _____
Osteoporosis	_____	Family member(s) _____
Thyroid Disease	_____	Family member(s) _____
Autoimmune Disease	_____	Family member(s) _____

Allergies: Please check all that apply.

_____ penicillin   _____ morphine   _____ dye allergies   _____ pet allergies

_____ codeine   _____ aspirin   _____ nitrate allergy   _____ seasonal (pollen)

_____ sulfa drugs   _____ food allergies _____ no known allergies   other: _____

Please describe the allergic reaction you experienced and when it occurred?

_____

_____

_____

Current Prescription Medications:

Medication Name	Strength	Date Started	How often per day

List Hormones previously taken.	Date Started	Date Stopped	Reason Stopped

Patient Name (please print): _____

Over-the-counter (OTC) issues:

Please check all products that you use occasionally or regularly. Check all that apply.

Pain Reliever/anti-inflammatory:

_____ Aspirin

_____ Acetaminophen

_____ Ibuprofen

_____ Naproxen

_____ Other

Combination Cold Products:

_____ Cough Suppressant

_____ Antihistamine product

_____ Decongestant product

_____ Combination cold product

Other:

_____ Sleep aid

_____ Antidiarrheal

_____ Laxatives/stool softeners

_____ Diet aids/weight loss products

_____ Antacid

_____ Acid Blocker

_____ Other (please list)

_____

_____

_____

Supplements: Please identify and list the products you are using:

☐ vitamins (examples: multiple or single vitamins such as B complex, E, C, beta carotene)

_____

☐ minerals (examples: calcium, magnesium, chromium, etc.)

_____

☐ herbs (examples: Ginseng, Ginko Biloba, Echinacea, other herbal medicinal teas, tinctures, remedies, etc.)

_____

☐ enzymes (examples: digestive formulas, papaya, bromelain)

_____

☐ nutrition/protein supplements (examples: protein powders, amino acids, fish oils, etc.)

_____

☐ others, please list: _____

_____

_____

Patient Name (please print):_____

List use of:			Qty.	Daily	Weekly	Monthly	Occasionally
Tobacco?	□ NO	□ YES	_____	□	□	□	□
Alcohol?	□ NO	□ YES	_____	□	□	□	□
Caffeine?	□ NO	□ YES	_____	□	□	□	□

Have you ever used oral contraceptives: □ No   □ Yes

If yes, did you experience any problem(s)?   □ No   □ Yes

If YES, describe any problem(s).

_____

_____

_____

Do you have, or did you ever have Premenstrual Syndrome (PMS)?   □ No   □ Yes

If yes, please explain:

_____

_____

_____

Since you first began having periods, have you ever had what you would consider to be abnormal cycles?   ☐ No   ☐ Yes

If YES, please explain (such as age when this occurred, symptoms…):

_____

_____

_____

_____

_____

When was your last period? _____

How many days did it last? _____

Have you ever had fibrocystic breasts?   ☐ No   ☐ Yes

If yes, please explain (such as age when this occurred, symptoms, treatments…):

_____

_____

_____

Patient Name (please print):_____

Have you ever had uterine fibroids?   □ No   □ Yes

If yes, please explain (such as age when this occurred, symptoms, treatments…):

_____

_____

_____

_____

How many pregnancies have you had?_____   How many children?_____

Any interrupted pregnancies?   □ No   □ Yes

Have you had a hysterectomy?   □ No   □ Yes (date: _____)

Ovaries removed?   □ No   □ Yes (date: _____)

Have you had a tubal ligation?   □   No   □ Yes (date: _____)

Have you had any of the following tests performed? Check those that apply and note date of last test.

Mammography   □ No   □ Yes   Date: _____

PAP Smear   □ No   □ Yes   Date: _____

Patient Self-Assessment Symptom Evaluation

Please rate each of the following symptoms

	Absent	Mild	Moderate	Severe
Memory lapse	_____	_____	_____	_____
Foggy thinking	_____	_____	_____	_____
Bone loss	_____	_____	_____	_____
Incontinence	_____	_____	_____	_____
Increased urinary urge	_____	_____	_____	_____
Heart palpitations	_____	_____	_____	_____
Rapid heart beat	_____	_____	_____	_____
Hot flashes	_____	_____	_____	_____
Night sweats	_____	_____	_____	_____
Vaginal dryness/atrophy	_____	_____	_____	_____
Vaginal/Urinary Tract infections	_____	_____	_____	_____
Sleep disturbances/insomnia	_____	_____	_____	_____
Weight gain — waist	_____	_____	_____	_____
Weight gain — hips	_____	_____	_____	_____
Bleeding cycle changes	_____	_____	_____	_____
Breakthrough bleeding	_____	_____	_____	_____

	Absent	Mild	Moderate	Severe
Cramps	_____	_____	_____	_____
Fluid retention	_____	_____	_____	_____
Breast tenderness	_____	_____	_____	_____
Mood swings	_____	_____	_____	_____
Irritability	_____	_____	_____	_____
Nervousness	_____	_____	_____	_____
Anxiety	_____	_____	_____	_____
Infertility issues	_____	_____	_____	_____
Emotional instability	_____	_____	_____	_____
Decreased libido	_____	_____	_____	_____
Harder to reach climax	_____	_____	_____	_____
Decreased muscle size/strength	_____	_____	_____	_____
Decreased stamina	_____	_____	_____	_____
Loss of scalp hair	_____	_____	_____	_____

Patient Name (please print): _____

Patient Self-Assessment Symptom Evaluation, cont'd

	Absent	Mild	Moderate	Severe
Increased facial or body hair	_____	_____	_____	_____
Acne	_____	_____	_____	_____
Aches and pains	_____	_____	_____	_____
Stress	_____	_____	_____	_____
High blood pressure	_____	_____	_____	_____
Rapid aging	_____	_____	_____	_____
Cravings for sweets	_____	_____	_____	_____
Cravings for salt	_____	_____	_____	_____
Caffeine or nicotine needs	_____	_____	_____	_____
Allergies	_____	_____	_____	_____
Sensitivity to chemicals	_____	_____	_____	_____
Slow pulse rate	_____	_____	_____	_____
Low blood sugar	_____	_____	_____	_____
Low blood pressure	_____	_____	_____	_____
	Absent	Mild	Moderate	Severe

Morning fatigue　　　　　　　＿＿＿＿　　＿＿＿＿　　＿＿＿＿　　＿＿＿＿

Evening fatigue　　　　　　　＿＿＿＿　　＿＿＿＿　　＿＿＿＿　　＿＿＿＿

Headaches　　　　　　　　　＿＿＿＿　　＿＿＿＿　　＿＿＿＿　　＿＿＿＿

Depression　　　　　　　　　＿＿＿＿　　＿＿＿＿　　＿＿＿＿　　＿＿＿＿

Low (cold) body temperature　＿＿＿＿　　＿＿＿＿　　＿＿＿＿　　＿＿＿＿

Cold extremities　　　　　　　＿＿＿＿　　＿＿＿＿　　＿＿＿＿　　＿＿＿＿

Sensitivity to cold　　　　　　＿＿＿＿　　＿＿＿＿　　＿＿＿＿　　＿＿＿＿

High cholesterol　　　　　　　＿＿＿＿　　＿＿＿＿　　＿＿＿＿　　＿＿＿＿

Elevated triglycerides　　　　＿＿＿＿　　＿＿＿＿　　＿＿＿＿　　＿＿＿＿

Swelling of ankles/wrists　　　＿＿＿＿　　＿＿＿＿　　＿＿＿＿　　＿＿＿＿

Puffy eyes/face　　　　　　　＿＿＿＿　　＿＿＿＿　　＿＿＿＿　　＿＿＿＿

Dry or brittle hair　　　　　　＿＿＿＿　　＿＿＿＿　　＿＿＿＿　　＿＿＿＿

Brittle or breaking nails　　　　＿＿＿＿　　＿＿＿＿　　＿＿＿＿　　＿＿＿＿

Constipation　　　　　　　　＿＿＿＿　　＿＿＿＿　　＿＿＿＿　　＿＿＿＿

Dry skin　　　　　　　　　　＿＿＿＿　　＿＿＿＿　　＿＿＿＿　　＿＿＿＿

Thinning skin　　　　　　　　＿＿＿＿　　＿＿＿＿　　＿＿＿＿　　＿＿＿＿

Goiter　　　　　　　　　　　＿＿＿＿　　＿＿＿＿　　＿＿＿＿　　＿＿＿＿

Decreased sweating　　　　　＿＿＿＿　　＿＿＿＿　　＿＿＿＿　　＿＿＿＿

Hearing loss　　　　　　　　＿＿＿＿　　＿＿＿＿　　＿＿＿＿　　＿＿＿＿

Patient Name (please print):_____

When did your symptoms start?_____

Please describe any changes in symptoms associated with any hormone replacement or dosage changes:

_____

_____

_____

_____

_____

_____

Where did you receive the information to consider Bio-identical Hormone Restoration Therapy?

☐ Doctor   ☐ Friend/Family Member   ☐ Book   ☐ Other: _____

If by book, please list name and author of book: _____

What are your goals with taking BHRT?

_____

_____

_____

_____

_____

_____

Please write down any questions you have about Bio-identical Hormone Restoration Therapy:

_____

_____

_____

_____

_____

_____

_____

_____

_____

_____

_____

_____

_____

_____

Appendix C
Symptom Lists

High Cortisol Symptoms

Common Symptoms

Sleep disturbances	Bone Loss	Weight gain –abdomen, waist
Low libido	Anxiety	Mild depression
Hair loss (general or clumping)	Memory loss	Inflammation
Elevated triglycerides	Aches & pains	Wired but tired feeling

Symptoms of estrogen deficiency including hot flashes, night sweats, irregular cycles, headaches

Symptoms of progesterone deficiency including infertility, PMS symptoms, irregular (excessive) menses

Symptoms of testosterone deficiency including decreased sex drive, hyperemotional states, muscle weakness

Symptoms of hypothyroidism

Additional Symptoms

Irritability	Muscle weakness	Increased cholesterol
Foggy thinking	Confusion	Nervousness
Decreased muscle size	Increased bruising	Binge eating
Elevated blood pressure	Increase in infections	
Increased blood sugar	Increased insulin and insulin resistance	

Low Cortisol Symptoms

Common Symptoms

Cravings for salt, stimulants (sugar, caffeine, nicotine, carbohydrates), and high fat foods

Symptoms of hypothyroidism	Symptoms of low progesterone/estrogen dominance	
Fatigue (prolonged)	Allergies	Chemical sensitivities
Irritability	Decreased stamina	Poor memory & concentration
Feelings of being overwhelmed	Emotional instability	Lethargy
Mental fatigue	Apathy	

Additional Symptoms

Loss of motivation or initiative	Confusion	
Depression	Orthostatic hypotension	Low blood pressure
Hypoglycemia	Digestive problems	Heartburn
Low libido	Decreased sexual interest	Decreased athletic performance
Poor healing of wounds	Decreased immune function / increased infections	
Increased drug use	Increased alcohol intake	Chloasma (liver spots)
Decreased ability to handle stress	Edema	Dizziness
Sensitivity to light	Aches & pain	

Note: Symptoms of both high and low cortisol coexist under chronic stress and indicate adrenal dysfunction

Female Symptom Lists

Estrogen Deficiency Symptoms

Common Symptoms

Hot flashes	Night sweats	Heart palpitations
Sleep disturbances	Memory loss/lapses	Foggy thinking
Low libido	Vaginal dryness/atrophy	Painful intercourse
Bone loss	Headaches	Depression
Vaginal & bladder infections	Weight gain (waist)	Dry Skin

Additional Symptoms

Anxiety	Emotional instability	Elevated blood pressure
Incontinence	Increase in urinary urge	UTIs
Decreased verbal skills	Poor concentration	Hair loss
Increased wrinkles	Thinning skin	Acne/oily skin
Difficult to lose weight	Food cravings	Aches and pains
Decreased breast size	Dry eyes	

Estrogen Dominance (excess estrogen or high estrogen relative to progesterone)

Common Symptoms

Symptoms of estrogen deficiency (due to down-regulation of estrogen receptors)

Breast swelling and tenderness	Fibrocystic breasts	Uterine fibroids/cysts
Cravings for sweets	Weight gain (abdomen, hips, & thighs)	Fatigue
Nervousness	Anxiety	Irritability
Mood swings	Fluid retention	Heavy irregular menses
PMS symptoms	Low thyroid symptoms	Headaches

Additional Symptoms

Bloating	Low libido	Decreased sexual interest
Gall bladder problems	Blood sugar problems	Sleep disturbances
Cervical dysplasia	Depression with anxiety or agitation	

Female Symptom Lists

Progesterone Deficiency

Common Symptoms

Symptoms of estrogen excess (relative lack of progesterone)

Swollen or tender breasts	Irregular menses (usually excessive)	PMS symptoms
Cramping	Weight gain	Infertility
Depression	Anxiety	Fuzzy thinking
Acne/oily skin	Joint pain	Headache

Additional Symptoms

Low libido	Uterine fibroids	Insomnia
Mood swings	Irritability	Nervousness
Osteoporosis	Inflammation	Hair loss
Low thyroid symptoms	Decreased HDL levels	

Migraines/headaches prior to menstrual cycles

Progesterone Excess

Common Symptoms

Exacerbates symptoms of estrogen deficiency (down-regulation of estrogen receptors)

Somnolence	Drowsiness	Mild depression
Gastrointestinal bloating	Breast swelling	Candida exacerbations

Additional Symptoms

Increased infections --suppressed immune system   Incontinence (leaky bladder)

Back, leg and hip aches (causes ligaments to relax excessively)

Decreased glucose tolerance	Increased insulin resistance	Increased fat storage

Decreased growth hormone   Increased appetite (carbohydrate cravings)

Bloating/constipation (relaxes smooth muscle of the gut)   Increased cortisol

Female Symptom Lists

Testosterone Deficiency

Common Symptoms

Fatigue (prolonged)	Memory lapse	Mental fuzziness
Muscle weakness/wasting	Heart palpitations	Bone loss
Decreased libido	Vaginal dryness/atrophy	Incontinence
Depression	Diminished feeling of well-being	Blunted motivation
General aches and pains	Dry, thinning skin with poor elasticity	Fibromyalgia

Additional symptoms

Anxiety	Hyperemotional states	Rapid aging
Weight gain	Decreased stamina	Deceased muscle tone
Headaches	Decreased sex drive	Low self-esteem
Allergies	Dry, thinning hair	Thin lips
Increased flatulence	Droopy eyelids	Saggy cheeks
Loss of pubic hair	Decreased dreaming	

Testosterone Excess

Common Symptoms

Acne or oily skin	Deepening of voice	Clitoral enlargement
Increased body hair	Scalp hair loss	Insomnia
Moodiness	Irritability	Anger
Hirsutisim	Aggressiveness	Agitation

Additional Symptoms

Depression	Anxiety	Increased insulin resistance
Hypoglycemia	Decreased HDL levels	Elevated triglycerides
Fatigue	Fluid retention	Infertility
Salt and sugar cravings	Weight gain (waist)	

Female Symptom Lists

DHEA Deficiency

Decreased energy	Muscle weakness	Irritability
Difficulties dealing with stress	Weight gain	Joint soreness
Decreased immune function – increase in infections		Rapid aging
Depression	Loss of hair (scalp, axial, pubic)	Anxiety
Low libido	Dry eye	Fatigue
Dry skin		

Symptoms of low testosterone and/or low estrogen due to less conversion from DHEA

DHEA Excess

Acne	Anger	Deepening of voice
Increased facial or body hair	Mild depression	Fatigue
Insomnia	Irritability	Mood changes
Restless sleep	Sugar cravings	Weight gain (waist)
Hair loss	Oily skin	Anxiety
Cardiac irregularities	Headaches	Elevated liver enzymes
Increased facial hair		

Symptoms of excess testosterone and/or estrogen due to increased conversion

Hyperthyroidism Symptoms

Weight loss	Excessive sweating	Heat intolerance
Chest pain	Heart racing	Mild depression
Anxiety	Irritability	Moodiness
Insomnia	Fatigue	Muscle weakness
Increased bowel movements	Loose stools or diarrhea	Hair loss
Light or absent menses	Shortness of breath	Staring gaze
Warm, moist skin	Puffiness around eyes	Thickening of skin of lower legs

Insulin Deficiency/Insulin Resistance Symptoms

Bone loss	Depression	Fatigue	Insomnia
Blurry vision	Increased urinary frequency	Excessive thirst	
Heart disease	Neuropathies	High blood pressure	
Slow wound healing	Numbness in feet and legs	Constant hunger	
Chronic infections (skin, gums, urinary tract)		High protein in urine	
Hyperglycemia	Weight loss	Genital itching (women)	

Insulin Excess Symptoms

High blood pressure	High cholesterol	High triglycerides
Weight gain	Elevated cortisol	Inflammation
Depression	Mood swings	Insomnia
Accelerated aging	Infertility	Migraine headaches
Osteopenia/osteoporosis	Heartburn	Irritable bowel syndrome
Asthma	Acne	Increased heart disease
Symptoms of estrogen deficiency		

Male Symptom Lists

Testosterone Deficiency Symptoms

Common Symptoms

Burned-out feeling	Apathy	Irritability
Fatigue	Decreased stamina	Sleep disturbances
Increased urinary urge	Decreased urinary flow	Depression
Decreased muscle mass	Night sweats	Weight gain (waist)
Erectile dysfunction	Decreased erections	Decreased libido/sex drive
Infertility issues	Mental fatigue	Prostate problems

Additional Symptoms

Hair loss (scalp & body)	Osteoporosis	Decreased bone density
Breast development	Moodiness	Loss of self esteem
Lack of motivation	Oily skin	Decreased mental sharpness
Fibromyalgia	Hot flashes	Inability to lose weight

Testosterone Excess Symptoms

Symptoms of testosterone deficiency (due to down-regulation of receptors)

Testicle Shrinkage	Enlarged prostate	High sex drive
Aggressiveness	Impulsiveness	Competitiveness
Insensitivity to others	Acne (primarily back & shoulder)	Hair loss

Weight gain, breast enlargement, moodiness -- from conversion to estrogen

Symptoms of Hypothyroidism (Hypometabolism)

Common Symptoms

Loss of energy (fatigue/malaise)	especially evening fatigue	Decreased stamina
Low body temperature	Cold intolerance/sensitivity	Cold extremities
Weight gain	Difficulty losing weight	Insomnia
Dry skin	Skin pallor, pastiness and puffiness	Thinning skin
Myxedema	Swollen, puffy eyes and eyelids	Fluid retention
Goiter/enlarged thyroid	Headaches	Constipation
High cholesterol	Elevated triglycerides	Decreased sweating
Depression	Mood Swings	Irritability
Memory lapse	Poor concentration	Decreased mental sharpness
Foggy thinking	Confusion	Forgetfulness
Brittle nails	Dry, brittle hair	Hair stops growing
Hair loss(scalp, diffuse)	Loss of outer (lateral) 1/3 of eyebrows	Hair loss (legs, arms, axillary)
Infertility	Recurrent miscarriages	Menstrual cycle irregularities
Low libido	Night sweats	Increase in hot flashes
Muscle & joint pain & cramps	Slowed reflexes and movements	Slowed speech
Low blood pressure	Slow pulse rate	Heart palpitations/fibrillations

Additional Symptoms

Sleep apnea	Gallstones	Allergies/hives
Decreased cardiac output	Poor circulation	Dizziness/vertigo
Fibromyalgia	Carpel Tunnel Syndrome	Morning stiffness
High insulin levels	Hypoglycemia	Appetite changes
Endometriosis	Uterine fibroids	Fibrocystic breasts
Decreased sex drive	Painful periods/PMS	Acne (face, scalp)
Anxiety/panic attacks	Lack of motivation	Muscle weakness
Recurrent or chronic infections	Mild elevation of liver enzymes	Elbow keratosis
Hearing loss	Sore throat	Hoarse, husky voice
Loss or thinning of eyelashes	Drooping eyelids	Dull facial expressions
Tinnitus	Excessive ear wax	Dry, itchy ear canals
Eye spasms	Turned down mouth	Yellow coloring of skin
Fat buildup at clavicle	Parathesias (tingling/numbness of extremities)	Bruising

BHRT Physiologic Dosing Guidelines (Females) – Bi-est 50:50

- Protocol is to give new BHRT patients the smallest effective starting dose.
- Compounding allows great flexibility in titrating doses to meet individual needs.
- *Note: Micronized hormones are used in the following:*

Condition	Hormone	Route	Dosage Range	Dosing	Days Given	Notes
PMS	Progesterone	Oral SR	25-400 mg daily (Usual 25-100 mg)	1-2 x daily	Cyclically days 14-25	May adjust days of therapy p.r.n.
		Topical	5-30 mg daily (Usual 5-20 mg)	1-2 x daily	Cyclically days 14-25	May adjust days of therapy p.r.n.
Peri-Menopause	Progesterone	Oral SR	25-400 mg daily (Usual 100-200 mg)	1-2 x daily	Cyclically days 14-25	May adjust days of therapy p.r.n.
		Topical	5-50 mg daily (Usual 20-30 mg)	1-2 x daily	Cyclically days 14-25	May adjust days of therapy p.r.n.
	Bi-estrogen (50:50)	Topical	0.05-0.20 mg daily (Start low and increase slowly)	1-2 x daily	Cyclically days 1-25	Continue Progesterone as above
Menopause (Natural or Post-Menopause)	Testosterone and DHEA	p.r.n.	see dose age recommendations below under menopause			

Same protocol as surgical menopause (below); may need less testosterone
Make sure progesterone to estrogen ratio is high enough to suppress endometrial hyperplasia
If patient/physician is not absolutely sure patient is no longer producing endogenous hormones, dose cyclically as in peri-menopause
If lack of menopausal symptoms, use lower end of dosage ranges and monitor BMD, Lipids, BP, cognitive function

Condition	Hormone	Route	Dosage Range	Dosing	Days Given	Notes
Menopause (Surgical)	Progesterone	Oral SR	25-400 mg daily (Usual 100-200 mg)	1-2 x daily	May use continuously	
		Topical	10-50 mg daily (Usual 20-30 mg)	1-2 x daily	Use 6 days per week	
	Bi-estrogen (50-50)	Topical	0.05-0.25 mg daily	1-2 x daily	May use continuously or 6 days per week	
	Testosterone	Oral SR	1.0-4.0 mg daily	1x daily in a.m.		
		Topical	0.25-2.0 mg daily	1x daily in a.m.		
	DHEA (optional)	Oral SR	5-20 mg daily (Usual 5-10 mg)	1x daily in a.m.		
		Topical	0.5-2.5 mg daily	1x daily in a.m.		Note: Oral estradiol is not recommended because (1) high level of estrone produced and (2) oral estrogens are not as safe as other routes of administration
Cancer Risk Patients	Estriol	Oral SR	0.5-8 mg daily	1-2 x daily		
		Topical/vaginal	0.1-2 mg daily (Usual 0.25-0.5mg)	1-2 x daily	Titrate up until symptoms become tolerable; monitor BMD, Lipids, BP	

Note: Sublingual total daily doses are usually twice those of topical when administered as b.i.d. dosing; dose 25-33% total daily dosage less than this if administered as t.i.d. dosing. (Example: progesterone in menopause, sublingually 50 mg b.i.d or 20-25mg t.i.d)

Please note: Dosing guidelines are meant to be used as a reference only. They are in no way indicating a recommendation for any product, for any patient, or for any clinical situation. Individual dosage should be determined based on results of a hormone/total health evaluation for each patient. Dosages given are the opinion of the author based on his experiences.

BHRT Physiologic Dosing Guidelines (Male)

Note: <u>Micronized hormones are used in the following:</u>

Protocol is to give new BHRT patients the smallest effective starting dose.

Hormone	Route	Dosage Range (daily unless noted)	Dosing	Notes
Testosterone	S/L or Buccal	2.5 to 20 (usual 5-10)	2-3 times per day	Allow to dissolve under tongue or in buccal pouch. Do not swallow
	Topical cream/lotion	1 to 20 mg (usual 5-10)	Once (a.m.) or twice daily	Non-penetrating base. Rub in well. Wash hands prior to and after use. Caution on possibility of transfer
	IM injection	50 to 80 mgs weekly	Weekly	Cypionate or enanthate
	Implantable Pellets	4 to 6 x 200 mg pellets	q 6 months	
DHEA	Oral	5 to 25 mg	Daily in a.m.	IR or SR
	S/L or buccal	2.5 to 15 mg	2 times daily	Allow to dissolve under tongue or in buccal pouch, Do not swallow
	Topical cream/lotion	1 to 10 mg	Daily in a.m.	Non-penetrating base. Rub in well. Wash hands prior to and after use. Caution on possibility of transfer
Progesterone	Oral	5-20 mg (usual 5-10)	Once Daily h.s.	SR capsule
	Topical cream/lotion	0.25-2.5 mg (usual 1-2)	Once daily	Non-penetrating base. Rub in well. Wash hands prior to and after use. Caution on possibility of transfer
	S/L or buccal	2.5 to 10 mg (usual 2.5 to 5)	2-3 times per day	Allow to dissolve under tongue or in buccal pouch, Do not swallow
Pregnenolone	Oral	10-100 mg (usual 25-50)	IR or SR, 1-2 x daily	
	Topical	1-10 mg (usual 2-5 mg)	Once daily	Non-penetrating base. Rub in well. Wash hands prior to and after use. Caution on possibility of transfer
Aromatase Inhibition				
Arimidex	Oral	0.5 to 1.0 mg	q.o.d. to b.i.w.	
Aromasin	Oral	25 mg	2-3 times per week	
Aromat8-PN (Xymogen)		80mg	1-2 capsules daily	
Chrysin	Oral	500-3000mg (usual 500-1500)	1-3 times daily	Pharmaceutical grade
Chrysin	Topical cream/lotion	30-50 mg	daily	Compounded

Note: Must correct underlying adrenal dysfunction, thyroid deficiency, and nutritional deficiency first or concurrently for hormones to provide expected symptom relief

Confidential Thyroid Hormone Evaluation

Today's Date: _____ / _____ / _____

Name: _____ DOB: _____ / _____ / _____ Age: _____

Address: _____

City, State, Zip: _____

Phone: Day: _____ Evening: _____

E-mail Address: _____

Gender: Male _____ Female _____ Height: _____ Wt: _____

Current Physicians:

Name Address Phone Number

_____

_____

_____

_____

Social History:

Have you ever used tobacco? If so, how often and how much? _____

Have you ever used alcohol? If so, how often and how much? _____

Do you use caffeine? If so, how often and how much? _____

Do you exercise? If so, what type, how long, how often? _____

Medical History:

Please list any allergies: (medication, pet, seasonal, food, dyes) _____

_____

Please describe the allergic reaction you experienced and when it occurred: _____

_____

Do you take any over-the-counter medications, nutritional or protein supplements
(including SOY), or herbal/homeopathic medications and list for what reason: _____

_____

_____

_____

Medical Conditions/Diseases: Please check all that apply.

_____ Cardiovascular (heart failure, heart attack)	_____ Arthritis
_____ Hyperlipidemia (elevated cholesterol or lipids)	_____ Depression
_____ Hypertension (high blood pressure)	_____ Epilepsy
_____ Cancer	_____ Ulcers
_____ Hyperthyroid	_____ Diabetes
_____ Hypothyroid	_____ Lung disorders
_____ Asthma, emphysema, COPD or other	_____ Stroke
_____ Blood clotting problems	
_____ Anemia (iron deficiency)	
_____ Hormonal related issues	

Do you have a history of whiplash or other neck injuries? If so, please describe and include date occurred. _____

_____

_____

Are you currently taking: Please circle all that apply.

Amiodarone (Cordarone®)	Carbamazepine (Tegretol®)
Levo/Carbidopa (Sinemet®)	Androgens (Testosterone, DHEA)
Danocrine (Danazol®)	Phenytoin (Dilantin®)
Metoclopramide (Reglan®)	Lithium
Estrogens (patch, tablets, topical, oral contraceptives)	Cholestyramine (Questran®, Prevalite®)
Glucorticoids (hydrocortisone, prednisone, prednisolone, etc.)	

Current Prescription Medications:

Medication Name	Strength	#Per Day	Date Began

PATIENT SELF-ASSESSMENT

SYMPTOMS	ABSENT	MILD	MODERATE	SEVERE
Depression				
Weight gain				
Cold extremities				
Cold intolerance				
Feel chilly				
Dry hair				
Brittle hair				
Dry skin				
Eczema				
Acne				
Puffy eyelids, face				
Brittle nails				
Menorrhagia				
Constipation				
Mentally sluggish				
Headache				
Insomnia				
Early morning fatigue				
Late morning fatigue				
Evening fatigue				
Muscle cramps				
Low sex drive				

When did symptoms start? _____

_____

_____

Any family history of ANY thyroid diseases? Please list whom and what type
(goiter, hypothyroidism, hyperthyroidism, Graves' Disease, Hashimoto's Disease).

_____

_____

Have you ever been tested for thyroid problems? Please list doctor, when
diagnosed, and any therapy given. _____

_____

_____

Do you have any current lab results (TSH, T4, Free T4,T3, Free T3, rT3, Lipid
panel, Hemoglobin, Iron, etc.)? Please provide documentation.

_____

_____

Have you had any other additional thyroid tests performed? _____

_____

_____

DISCLAIMER: By signing this form, I authorized the release of my medical
information to share with other healthcare professionals for treatment purposes
only.

      _____
      Signature

Appendix F
Basal Body Temperature

The "basal body temperature" test was developed by Broda O. Barnes, M.D. almost 60 years ago. Because thyroid hormone is so vital to cellular metabolism, reduced thyroid function most often manifests as a drop in body temperature to below the normal level of 98.6° F.

Some practitioners feel it is better to use a basal thermometer, which is more accurate than a regular oral thermometer. A basal thermometer for this purpose may be more accurate than any digital electronic thermometer. Dr. Barnes suggested that the temperature not be taken orally, but instead under the arm, with the person lying quietly in bed and the arm comfortably at the side. The temperature is taken upon awakening, before rising up out of the bed for any reason.

How to Check the Basal Body Temperature:

- Have thermometer within arm's reach upon going to bed

- Use a basal thermometer or a digital thermometer

- Immediately upon awakening, and with as little movement a possible, place thermometer under the arm

- Leave thermometer under the arm for 10 minutes or until indicator sounds

- Record the readings on three consecutive days (Dr. Barnes recommends 10 consecutive days, but most practitioners that use this test require an average over three days). Record date and temperature.

- Non-menstruating women, men, and children can test at any time. Menstruating women begin the temperature measurements on day 2 or day 3 of their cycle.

Normal axillary temperature is 97.8°-98.2° F. If the average temperature is less than 97.8°, then according to Dr. Barnes, the patient may have hypothyroidism. A low body temperature indicates suboptimal metabolism, which is most commonly caused by suboptimal thyroid function.

Low grade infections can raise body temperature resulting in normal or above basal body temperature. If symptoms of hypothyroidism exist, once low grade infection is adequately addressed, temperature should be retested.

Dr. Barnes felt that this test was a check on the most basic function of the thyroid gland: its ability to regulate the metabolic furnace of the body, and to control temperature. An average of three or ten days is a very useful indication, therefore, of one's overall thyroid status and, in many people, may well be more accurate in indicating low thyroid function than conventional serum thyroid tests. Temperature testing, as with all testing, is not infallible, and should never be used alone to diagnose or rule out a thyroid condition, or to dictate therapy. This test is simply a good piece of information that should be used wisely.

A low basal body temperature indicates low metabolism, but does not give information as to where the cause or causes of low metabolism are occurring. Functional thyroid testing should be done to evaluate possible causes.

References

- Broda A Barnes M.D. and Lawrence Galton. <u>Hypothyroidism: The Unsuspected Illness</u>. New York,: Harper and Row, 1976
- David Brownstein, M.D. <u>Overcoming Thyroid Disorders</u>. Medical Alternative Press, 2008

Appendix G
Approaches to Autoimmune Reactions

1) Eliminate the agent or agents initiating the reaction

- Elimination diet -

  - Eliminate gluten 100% for at least 60 days. Reevaluate based on symptom improvements and changes in TPO or TgAb levels. The antigen for gluten appears to be cross sensitive for the antigen for TPO and possibly the antigen for TG, therefore gluten is a common source of thyroid autoimmune reactions.

    - If partial improvement, continue gluten free diet, and eliminate dairy also or do food sensitivity testing (ALCAT)

  OR

  - Do food sensitivity testing before initiating an elimination diet

  OR

  - Dr. Alan Gaby recommends a modified form of the elimination diet recommended by William Crook, M.D. This diet removes all common allergens including wheat (oats, barley, & rye allowed so it is *not gluten free*), dairy, eggs, corn, citrus fruits, coffee, tea, alcohol, refined sugars, any known allergens, any food the patient eats three or more times a week, and artificial colors, flavors, preservatives, sweeteners, and texturing agents. After symptoms improve in two to three weeks, foods are added back to the diet one at a time to see if there is then a response. If you wish to follow this elimination diet, details can be provided. If you do follow this diet, we recommend that you eliminate gluten also.

  - Note: Diet should be low glycemic index too. Small more frequent meals if possible. Patient should keep a food diary.

  - Remove artificial sweeteners

  - Remove trans fats, aspartame, and processed whole foods from diet

2) Heavy Metal Testing   (DMSA challenge test with Doctors Data, Metagenix, Genova)

3) Selenium 400 mcg (daily total, including what patient may be taking in MVM, thyroid support, and adrenal

support products)

4) Magnesium 600mg as magnesium glycinate (total daily dose)

5) Reduce gut inflammation and restore normal GI flora

- Anti-inflammatory diet

- Probiotic

- Medicinal food for healthy gut and to decrease inflammation (Metagenics and others) and L-Glutamine

6) Treat any underlying infections, including mycoplasma infections. May want to consider stool test for parasites and viruses (Genova and others)

7) Correct any underlying hormone deficiencies & imbalances, especially low DHEA and adrenal dysfunction

8) Best to avoid use of any glandular products, and supplement iodine with caution

9) May wish to attempt to restore TH-1 and TH-2 balance (See "Why Do I Still Have Thyroid Symptoms? When My Lab Tests Are Normal" by Datis Kharrazian

Appendix H
Iodine Testing and Supplementation Guidelines

Iodine testing should not be done in urine. Serum iodine is of little value in that it does not represent intracellular levels and saliva testing may be difficult to interpret due to a lack of valid reference ranges. Urine testing can be done in three ways:

- 24-hour urine collection following a loading dose of 50 mg of iodine. Some labs use a 90% excretion rate as normal. Normal dietary iodine intake is 90% excreted in 24 hours, but a dose of 50 mg may take up to 48 hours to be 90% eliminated. Be sure to evaluate results on a normal 24-hour excretion of a 50 mg loading dose as 60-70% excretion.
  - Cost at time of printing was $90 and higher for several laboratories
- Dried Urine testing. Morning and last void of the day are collected for dipping a strip, and the dried strips are mailed to the lab. Normal range is based on WHO criteria and additional data. Patients should be at a high normal to slightly high level.
  - Cost at time of printing was $70 (ZRT Laboratory)
- Random spot urine testing. This is not of much use in itself since iodine levels vary with diet and time of day, and no reference range would be applicable.

Dosing of Iodine

Iodine can be dosed based on a measurement indicating a low level, or on a trial basis in a patient with hypothyroid symptoms. Daily requirement of iodine for production of thyroid hormone is approximately 150 mcg, but additional iodine may be needed for optimal symporter function, proper iodination of lipids in the thyroid gland, and protective benefits of iodine on breast, ovarian, and prostate cells. The optimal level of iodine, and therefore optimal dosing, in any individual has not been established.

Administration of 150 mcg to 1.0 mg daily should supply sufficient iodine for thyroid hormone production in the average patient. However, higher doses of up to 25 to 50 mg daily have provided good clinical response in some individuals. Clinically, many patients show improvement in symptoms with a small amount of iodine. Some improve more with increasing doses, and some may start to experience a worsening of symptoms at a higher dose, and then improvement when dose is lowered again.

Initial dosage of iodine should be conservative, at 375 mcg to 500 mcg daily. Increase dosage slowly, every 3-4 weeks. If improvements are seen with an increase, dose can continued to be increased every few weeks. If no improvements are seen, continue maintenance at present dose. If patient's symptoms worsen, decrease to and maintain at previous dose.

Note: You may use kelp or similar products to provide small amounts of iodine as long as the product is standardized to iodine content.

Note: Iodine supplementation may initially increase TSH level. TSH stimulates the NaI transporter, the mechanism by which iodine is transported within the cell. When iodine levels are low, TSH decreases somewhat. When iodine is supplemented in someone with low iodine levels, TSH will rise to increase absorption of iodine.

Note: Iodine supplementation may cause an increase in the level of TPO antibodies. In a patient with a high TPO antibody level and low iodine, address the autoimmune reaction, supplement with a good antioxidant combination (i.e., resveratrol and NAC) for 1-2 months Once TPO antibody level is decreasing, add iodine slowly and monitor TPO antibody level.

Appendix I
Thyroid Gradient Levels

Thyroid Gradient Levels

The Thyroid Gradient Level diagrams are used to compare selected results. Results are graphed on the diagram and lines drawn that can be described as hands on the face of a clock. If thyroid binding and conversion are all "normal," then all results would point in the same direction within their individual ranges.

Production

TT4 is the best indication of thyroid hormone production from the thyroid gland.

Extent of Binding

Comparing fT4 to TT4 provides an indication of binding (TBG)

If fT4 is lower within its normal range *relative to* where TT4 is within its normal range, this would indicate more than the normal amount of binding. For example, fT4 result was "12:00 o'clock" and TT4 result was "2:00 o'clock", this would indicate more binding than normal (even though fT4 would be optimal). Excessive binding can be caused by any relative excessive estrogen state, but most commonly by oral estrogen replacement therapy or by oral and/or excessive thyroid replacement therapy.

Note: binding proteins can change slowly over a period of several months as a result of any change in therapy affecting the binding protein. Follow-up testing should not be done for at least 90 days following initiation or any change in thyroid or oral estrogen therapy.

Conversion of T4 to T3

Comparing fT3 to fT4 provides interpretation as to the conversion of T4 to the active T3.

Example: If fT3 result was at "10:00 o'clock" on the dial, and fT4 result was at "12:00 o'clock", fT3 would be low *relative to* the fT4. This would indicate a less than normal rate of conversion.

Additionally, comparing fT3 to rT3 also provides information as to how T4 is being converted. fT3 and rT3 are normally produced in approximately equal amounts from T4, and the results within their respective ranges should be the same (i.e.: clock hands should point in the same direction).

If rT3 is higher within its range *relative to* fT3, the T4 is being converted to rT3 greater than normally occurs and less to T3 as normally occurs. The excess reverse T3 blocks the effects of lower than normal amount of fT3.

rT3 testing is most often outsourced, resulting in a longer time to get test results. rT3 testing involves radioactive material, so therefore is expensive and not earth-friendly. Since information on conversion can be obtained by comparing the fT3 level to the fT4 level, reverse T3 testing should not be a first choice and should be reserved for follow up testing in difficult patients.

Occasionally the fT3 level is high *relative to* the fT4 level. Since fT3 is normally produced from fT4 as needed, this situation would most likely indicate (1) an autoimmune reaction that is skewing the results, (2) the patient was not at complete rest prior to sampling, or (3) patient is in the initial phases of iodine deficiency and the body is maintaining a higher level of T3 in response to lack of production.

Note: Any test results compared must be obtained at exactly the same time using the same lab.

Note: Patient needs to be at complete rest for *at least* 15 minutes prior to obtaining blood sample.

Thyroid Gradient Levels

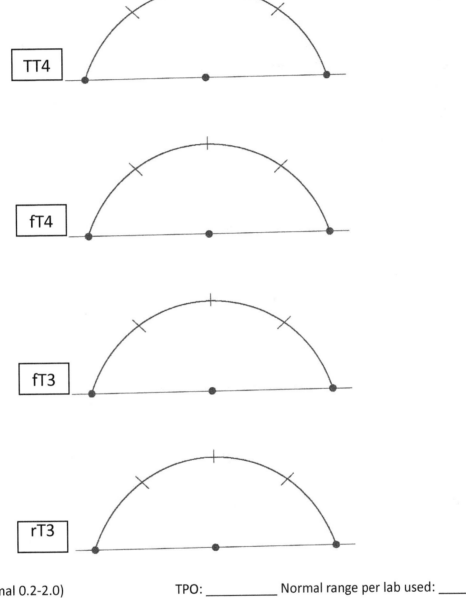

TSH: _____ (Optimal 0.2-2.0)   TPO: _____ Normal range per lab used: _____

Basal body temperature (3 consecutive days): _____° _____° _____° Average: _____°

THRT: Type: _____ Dosage: _____ How often: _____ Last taken: _____

Vitamin D level: _____ Dose if taking: _____

Ferritin level: _____

Iodine level: _____ Normal range for testing lab used: _____

Was patient at complete rest for at least 15 minutes prior to obtaining blood sample? _____

Thyroid Gradient Levels, Example I

Female, Caucasian, age 37. Mother of two children, works part time

Chief symptoms: headaches, weight gain, mild depression, constipation, irregular cycling

No prescription medications, takes various OTC pain relievers for headaches. Eats healthy diet

Lab results indicate no issues with cortisol or sex steroids

Lab results from page 1:

- TT4 is 8.75 (normal 4.4-12.5, optimal 6.425-10.475)

- fT4 is 1.31 (normal 0.73-1.95, optimal 1.035-1.645)

- fT3 is 2.5 (normal 2.3-4.2, optimal 2.775-3.725)

- Vitamin D level is 42, ferritin level is 84

Interpretation:

- Average basal body temperature is 97.2°, indicating suboptimal metabolism

- TT4 is within optimal range, indicating good endogenous production of thyroid hormone from the gland

- fT4 is within optimal range, and very similar where it is within its range relative to where TT4 is within its range, indicating normal thyroid binding

- fT3 is less than optimal (although "normal"). Relative to fT4, fT3 is much lower within its range than where fT4 is within its range, indicating poor conversion of fT4 to fT3

- Ferritin is close to optimal for thyroid function (90-110) and most likely not contributing significantly to symptoms

- Vitamin D is within "normal" range, but less than needed for optimal thyroid function (at least 50-60)

Plan:

- Address poor conversion of fT4 to fT3:

    o Review causes of poor conversion and address as necessary, especially stress and cortisol

    o Basic supplementation includes daily MVM, selenium to a total of 400 mcg daily, zinc to a total of 50 mg daily and, if diabetic, chromium at 1,000 mcg daily.

- Supplement Vitamin D3 at 10,000 Units daily for 2-4 weeks, and then decrease to 5,000 Units daily. Retest level and adjust dosage if necessary in 2-3 months

Thyroid Gradient Levels, *Example I*

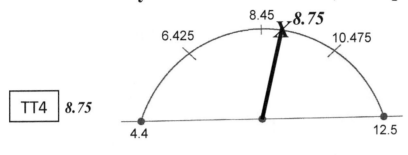

TT4 *8.75*

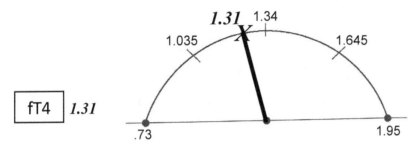

fT4 *1.31*

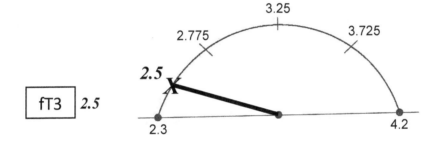

fT3 *2.5*

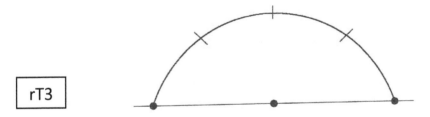

rT3

TSH: _____*2.4*_____ (Optimal 0.2-2.0)   TPO: _____*<10*_____ Normal range per lab used: _____*<10*_____

Basal body temperature (3 consecutive days): _*97.4*°_ _*97.0*°_ _*97.2*°_ Average: _*97.2*°_

THRT: Type: _____*N/A*_____ Dosage: _____ How often: _____ Last taken: _____

Vitamin D level: _____ Dose if taking: _*N/A*_____

Ferritin level: _____*84*_____

Iodine level: _____*UNK*_____ Normal range for testing lab used: _____

Was patient at complete rest for at least 15 minutes prior to obtaining blood sample? _____*UNK*_____

Thyroid Gradient Levels, Example II

Male, Caucasian, age 46, slightly overweight, teacher

Chief symptoms: fatigue, weight gain, headaches, depression, lethargy, decreased libido, general aches and pains

Takes Synthroid 150 mcg daily in a.m. OTC pain mediations

Hormone testing indicates high cortisol in morning and evening and low or low normal during day. Testosterone low normal for age.

Thyroid test results and interpretation:

- Average basal body temperature is low, indicating suboptimal metabolism

- TT4 is 13.9, higher than normal range. With last dose of T4 therapy taken 6 hours prior to blood sample, this indicates excessive T4 therapy

- fT4 is within optimal range, but compared to TT4, fT4 is lower within its range relative to where TT4 is within its range, indicating excessive binding

- fT3 is lower than optimal. Comparing to fT4, fT3 is much lower within its range relative to where fT4 is within its range, indicating poor conversion of fT4 to fT3.

- Vitamin D and ferritin are both lower than required for optimal thyroid function

Plan

- Gradually lower T4 dose while supporting function of thyroid gland and hormone
    - Lower T4 doses no more than 25% at one time, and retest no sooner than 90 days
    - Binding should decrease as T4 is decreased
- Address poor conversion of fT4 to fT3
    - Review causes of poor conversion and address as necessary, especially stress and cortisol
    - Basic supplementation includes daily MVM, selenium to a total of 400 mcg daily, zinc to a total of 50 mg daily and, if diabetic, chromium at 1,000 mcg daily.
- Supplement Vitamin D3 at 10,000 units daily for 4 weeks, then decrease to 5,000 Units daily. Retest level and adjust dosage if need in 2-3 months
- Supplement ferrous glycinate (or another well absorb chelated iron) at 50 mg of elemental iron daily for one week, then increase to 50 mg b.i.d. Retest level in 2-3 months. When optimal levels of ferritin are obtained, may reduce dosage to 15-25 mg daily.
- Test iodine levels on follow-up testing.

Thyroid Gradient Levels, *Example II*

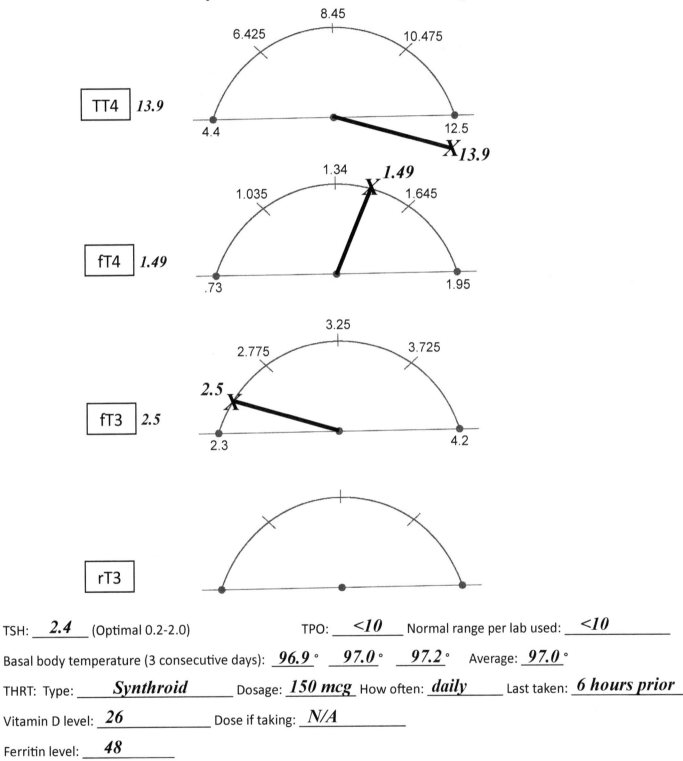

TSH: __*2.4*__ (Optimal 0.2-2.0)   TPO: __*<10*__ Normal range per lab used: __*<10*__

Basal body temperature (3 consecutive days): __*96.9*__° __*97.0*__° __*97.2*__°   Average: __*97.0*__°

THRT: Type: __*Synthroid*__   Dosage: __*150 mcg*__ How often: __*daily*__   Last taken: __*6 hours prior*__

Vitamin D level: __*26*__   Dose if taking: __*N/A*__

Ferritin level: __*48*__

Iodine level: __*UNK*__   Normal range for testing lab used: _____

Was patient at complete rest for at least 15 minutes prior to obtaining blood sample? __*YES*__

Appendix J
Thyroid Medication and Testing Interactions

Because of the possibility of decreased absorption, thyroid hormones should be administered on an empty stomach with a glass of water at least 30-60 minutes prior to food or enteral feedings. Antacids or mineral supplements containing aluminum, magnesium, iron, or calcium should be dosed at least 4 hours before or after thyroid medications. Thyroid hormones may administered in the morning or at night.

Foods that may inhibit absorption of thyroid hormones include:

Soybean flour, soy-based infant formulas or enteral feedings, high fiber diets, cottonseed meal, walnuts, and coffee.

Soy containing foods and soy isoflavones (genistein and daidzein) may interfere with thyroid peroxidase catalyzed iodination of thyroglobulin resulting in a decreased production of thyroid hormones and increase in TSH. Excessive soy may also interfere with the conversion of T4 to T3.

Drugs and supplements that decrease absorption of thyroid hormones:

Lithium, simethicone, cholestyramine (Questran®, Prevalite®), colestipol (Colestid®), sucralfate (Carafate®,Sulcrate®), sodium polystyrene sulfonate (Kayexalate), antacids, Sevelamer® (Renagel®), iron salts (including polysaccharide-iron complex), chromium, aluminum hydroxide, magnesium, calcium.

Drugs that decrease thyroid hormone function:

Amiodarone (Cordarone®) contains 37% iodine, inhibits conversion of T4 to T3 and is slowly eliminated. It can cause hyperthyroidism or hypothyroidism including life-threatening thyrotoxicosis. Abnormal thyroid function tests may persist for months after amiodarone discontinuation

Drugs containing bromide or fluoride can decrease the absorption of iodine leading to decreased thyroid function.

Drugs that **increase catabolism** of thyroid hormones (through hepatic enzyme induction):

Barbiturates, carbamazepine (Tegretol®), hydantoins, rifamycins, corticosteroids, didanosine (Videx®) chewable/dispersible tablets and oral powder for solution, raloxifene (Evista®).

Drugs that may increase TBG: estrogens (especially oral) and thyroid replacement, heroin, methadone,

5-fluorouracil, mitotane, tamoxifen

Drugs that may **inhibit conversion** of T4 to T3: glucocorticoids, beta blockers, SSRIs, antibiotics, lithium, opiates, phenytoin, theophylline, chemotherapy.

Drugs that increase thyroid hormone function:

Decrease metabolism of thyroid hormones: indinavir (IDV®, Crixivan®)

Drugs that may decrease TBG: androgens, anabolic steroids asparaginase (Elspar®), glucocorticoids (HC, prednisone,etc), phenytoin, salicylates, slow release nicotinic acid (Niaspan®)

Drugs that may reduce TSH secretion: Dopamine/Dopamine agonists, glucocorticoids, octreotide (Sandostatin®)

Drug Interactions

Thyroid hormone administration may:

• Necessitate adjustment of insulin or oral hypoglycemic agents. Blood glucose should be monitored when initiating or adjusting thyroid therapy in patients on these agents.

• Alter response to digoxin, requiring higher doses of digoxin.

• Increase the clearance of theophylline.

• Reduce effects of beta blockers

• Augment the response to anticoagulant medications (warfarin, heparin) or dicumarol. INRs should be monitored carefully in these patients.

• Increase effects of tricyclic antidepressants.

Sympathomimetic amines should be used with caution in patients with thyrotoxicosis as these patients are usually unusually responsive to these agents. Concomitant use of these agents with thyroid replacement can increase risk of coronary insufficiency.

Caution with co-administration of Ketamine; co-administration may cause marked hypertension and tachycardia.

References

Braverman L.E. and Utiger R.D.. Werner & Ingbar's The Thyroid, A Fundamental and Clinical Text. Lippincott Williams & Williams, Philadelphia PA. 2005

http://www.thyroidmanager.org/chapter/effects-of-the-environment-chemicals-and-drugs-on-thyroid-function/

Practitioner Pocket Guide to BHRT

Testing   (For further information see "Appropriate Hormone Testing" section)

- Females--initial testing (no supplementation)

    o Test estradiol (E2),progesterone (Pg), testosterone (T), DHEA or DHEAs (DS),and cortisol levels

        ▪ E and P can be tested in serum, capillary blood spot or saliva

        ▪ T and DHEA can be checked in blood spot or saliva (most serum labs do not use tests sensitive enough to be of clinical value)

        ▪ Cortisol should always be checked 4 point (4 times a day) in saliva

    o If symptoms of hypothyroidism: Test TT4, fT4, fT3, TSH, TPO, Vitamin D, and ferritin. (Iodine optional)

        ▪ Make sure to inform patient to be at complete rest for at least 15 minutes prior to sampling

- Females—follow up

    o Add estriol to above if supplementing estradiol or bi-est

    o See below on timing of dosing vs. timing of sample

- Males

    o E2, T, DS, SHBG, PSA, hematocrit, cortisol (4pt)   (progesterone optional)

        ▪ May alternatively measure both Total T and free T, then SHBG not required

    o T and DS can be tested in serum, capillary blood spot or saliva

    o Estradiol levels should be done in saliva or capillary blood

    o SHBG& PSA can be tested in serum or capillary blood spot

    o Hematocrit—serum

     o Cortisol—saliva

     o Hypothyroid symptoms – see above under female testing

     o On follow up testing, always monitor T, PSA, and hematocrit; others p.r.n.

<u>Timing of sample vs. timing of last dose prior to sampling:</u>

Oral SR dosage: Test 4-8 hours after last dose.

     If dosing b.i.d. test first thing in the morning, 8 hrs. after the last dose

     If dosing once daily, move dose the day before sample collection to evening, 8 hours prior to collection.

Topical administration

     Do not use serum testing with topical administration of hormones. Use saliva or blood spot testing from a lab with established reference ranges specific for topical administration

     Test levels at midpoint of dosing

          For patch, test near midpoint of duration of application

          For once daily application of creams, test 12 hours after last application

          For twice daily application, test 6-8 hours after last application

     Do not use saliva testing with sublingual or buccal administration. Use blood spot or serum. Test 4 hours after last dose if possible.

Dosing   (For more information see "Dosing Guidelines" and "Dosage Considerations" sections)

Females—usual starting doses as <u>total daily dose</u>

Progesterone   Oral SR(compounded)   PMS: 25-100mg   Peri-or Menopausal:100-200mg
May be given once daily at bedtime or b.i.d.

Topical cream   PMS: 5-20mg   Peri- or Menopausal: 20-30mg
May be dosed as once daily or twice a day

Sublingual or Buccal troches   PMS: 10-40mg   Peri- or Menopausal: 40-60mg
Dose at b.i.d or t.i.d.

Bi-est 50:50 (50% Estriol and 50% Estradiol)

Topical cream   0.05 to 0.10 mg daily to start.
May split into b.i.d. dosing if desired.

Sublingual or buccal   0.10 to 0.20 mg daily, b.i.d. dosage.
(0.075 to 0.15 total daily if t.i.d. dosing)

Testosterone   Topical cream   0.25 mg-2.0 mg daily in a.m. to start.
Maintenance dose is 0.1 to 0.5 mg daily.

DHEA   Oral IR   5-10mg daily.

Topical   0.5-2.0 mg daily

Pregnenolone   Oral SR: 10.0 to 20.0 mg   Topical: 1.0 to 2.0 mg

Males – usual starting doses as <u>total daily dose</u>

Testosterone	Topical cream/lotion	1.0 to 5.0 mg
	S/L or buccal troches	2.0 to 5.0 mg, one to two times daily
	IM injection	2.0 to 5.0 mg

Note: Aromatase inhibitor should be used if estrogen levels are high, or patient is overweight and/or stressed.

DHEA	Oral IR	5.0 to 25 mg
	S/L or buccal	5.0 to 10.0 mg, one to two times daily
	Topical	1.0 to 2.5 mg

Progesterone	Oral SR	5.0 to 10.0 mg
	Topical	0.5 to 1.0 mg
	S/L or buccal	1.0 to 2.0 mg, one to two times daily

Pregnenolone	Oral SR	10.0 to 20.0 mg
	Topical	1.0 to 2.0 mg

Example Prescriptions

Oral prescriptions: indicate SR and compounded:

1. Progesterone SR capsules 100mg compounded. #30 Take one capsule h.s.   2 refills.

Topical prescriptions:

Prescriber may indicate how much of a dose, and days supply, and months refills should cover, and pharmacist can determine quantities required:

1. Progesterone 20mg per dose topical cream

   Apply 20 mg twice a day to inside or arms and/or legs on days 14 through 25 of cycle.

   3 month supply with no refills.

2. Progesterone 20 mg per dose topical cream

   Apply 20 mg twice a day to inside or arms and/or legs for 4 weeks, and then decrease to 20mg applied once daily.

   1 month supply with refills for 2 months (or refill until "date")

Prescriber may want to be specific in quantity of cream to be applied and indicate days supply and let pharmacist determine quantity required.

1. Progesterone 20mg/0.25ml   100 day supply   No refill

   Apply 0.25ml (20 mg) to inside of arms and/or legs twice a day on days 14 through 2 of menstrual cycle.

2. Progesterone 20mg/0.25ml topical cream   I month supply (initially and refills)

   Apply 0.25 ml (20 mg) to inside of arms and/or legs twice a day for 4 weeks, then decrease to 0.25ml once a day.

   2 refills (or refill until "date").

Prescriber may want to indicate volume of dose as well as quantity.

1. Progesterone 20mg/0.25ml topical cream   15ml   1 refills

   Apply 0.25 ml (20 mg) to inside of arms and/or legs twice a day for 4 weeks, then decrease to 0.25ml once a day.

   (Note: 1 refill of 15 ml should last 60 days because dose will be 0.25 ml daily at time of refill.)

2. Progesterone 20mg/0.25ml   10 ml

   Apply 0.25ml (20 mg) to inside of arms and/or legs twice a day on days 14 through 2 of menstrual cycle.

   (Note: at 0.5 ml daily, at 12 days per month, 9 ml would be required to last 3 months.)

3. Bi-est: E2 0.05 mg and E3 0.05mg per 0.25ml in topical hormone cream base   15ml   1 refill

   Apply 0.25 ml (0.1mg) daily in the morning to inside of arm and/or leg 6 out of 7 days each week, skipping the same day each week.

Interpretation of thyroid levels and appropriate treatment options
(For complete explanation see the section on Hypothyroidism)

A high antibody level indicates an autoimmune response which is affecting the thyroid gland. This reaction can skew the other levels making the other issues listed below more difficult to analyze. Treatment for autoimmune issues is covered in a separate protocol, but the first step is to have the patient go on a 100% gluten-free diet for at least 60 days and retest.

If TT4 is less than optimal*then this indicates low production. Iodine and tyrosine are needed for production, as well as a number of vitamins. Treatment options include a good MVM such as Alpha Base by Ortho Molecular, assess tyrosine indicated in diet and supplement if low, and try a trail of iodine supplementation with kelp tablets, Lugol's iodine solution, or Iodoral tablets.

If ft4 is low *relative to* TT4 as indicated by the Thyroid Gradient Levels, excessive binding is occurring. Excessive binding is commonly caused by oral estrogen therapy, excessive thyroid therapy, or excessive estrogen (endogenous or supplemented). Treatment consists of removing causes and monitoring binding over time.

If ft3 is low *relative to* fT4, this indicates less than optimal conversion of T4 to T3. Factors adversely affecting conversion include stress, multiple mineral and vitamin deficiencies, alcohol abuse, medications, and more. See Dr. David Brownstein's book <u>Overcoming Thyroid Disorders</u> for a complete listing. Treatment options include a good MVM, selenium to a total of 300-400 mcg daily, zinc to a total of 25 to 50 mg daily, addressing stress including adaptogens to handle high or fluctuating cortisol levels.

Vitamin D level should be at least 60 for optimal thyroid receptor response.

Ferritin level should be 90-110 for optimal thyroid transport or utilization.

Cortisol levels need to be regulated, as high or low cortisol interferes with thyroid function in multiple levels.

Above treatment options should be followed for 2-3 months before retesting.

*optimal: take 25% of low end and high end of the lab's normal range to obtain the optimal range
   Example: normal for fT3 is 2.5 to 6.5. Optimal would be 3.5 to 5.5.

Adrenal Assessment and Treatment Options

With chronic stress, initially, high cortisol can result from an overactive HPA axis response. Eventually the ability to produce cortisol is reduced, leading to hypocortisolism.

Adrenal function can be addressed with lifestyle adaptations to stressors and stress response, nutritionals to regulate cortisol, vitamins and minerals specific to adrenal needs, and glandular products.

All patients with significant chronic stress can be treated with patient addressing stressors and stress response, adaptogens, and vitamin/mineral support.

High cortisol may be treated using adaptogens, and phosphatidylserine.

For patients with cortisol levels below normal, or at low-normal at least twice a day, in addition to adaptogens and an adrenal vitamin/mineral, treat with a glandular to help rebuild adrenal strength and reserves.

Adaptogens: Herbal Adrenal Support Formula by (Doctor Wilson's Original Formulations).
10-15 drops in juice or water 2-4 times daily
Adapten-All by Ortho Molecular   2 capsules 1-2 times daily

Phosphatidylserine (PS) 100mg: 1-3 capsules 2-3 hours prior to times of high cortisol. <u>Caution</u>: PS can further lower already low cortisol levels, so in patients with both high and low cortisol levels, suppression of high level use may increase fatigue during periods of low cortisol.

Adrenal vitamin/mineral: Super Adrenal Stress Formula (Doctor Wilson's Original Formulations): 1 caplet 3-5 times daily

Glandular: Adrenal Rebuilder (Doctor Wilson's Original Formulations): 1 caplet 3-6 times daily.

Printed in the USA
CPSIA information can be obtained
at www.ICGtesting.com
LVHW081150040524
779270LV00003B/43